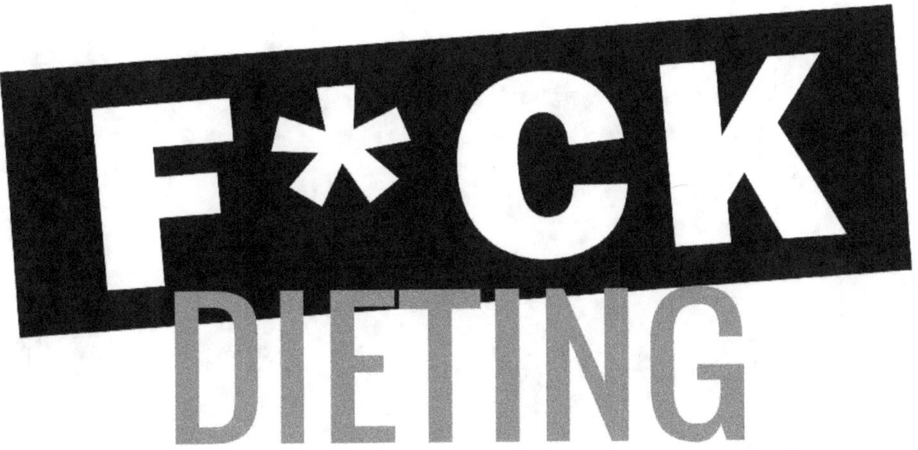

The Badass Guide to Smashing Diet Culture One F*cking Bite at a Time!

Logan West

Published by Clubhouse Publishing
This book is a work of non-fiction. While every effort has been made to ensure accuracy, the publisher and author make no warranties, express or implied, regarding the completeness, accuracy, or reliability of the information contained herein. The content is intended for entertainment and educational purposes only.

Table Of Contents

Diet Culture Can Kiss My Ass

Congratulations, you magnificent, food-loving badass—you just picked up the book that's about to change your relationship with food, your body, and all the ridiculous diet nonsense you've been fed (pun intended) your entire life. Let's be real: diets are the worst. They're like toxic exes—full of promises, short on delivery, and always leaving you feeling worse about yourself. But guess what? We're done with that shit.

Diet culture has been screwing with us for decades, whispering sweet lies about "clean eating," "guilt-free" snacks, and that mythical "summer body" we're all supposed to be chasing. It's convinced us that food is the enemy, that carbs are the devil, and that eating a cupcake is a moral failing. Meanwhile, it's raking in billions selling us celery juice and skinny teas while we cry over salad and secretly dream of fries. Well, fuck that.

Here's the truth: food is not the enemy. Your body is not a project to be fixed. And you are not a goddamn math equation of calories in and calories out. You're a human being, and food is one of life's greatest pleasures. It's meant to be enjoyed, not obsessed over. And that's what this book is all about—taking back your power, ditching the guilt, and learning to eat like the fabulous, unapologetic badass you are.

Now, let's talk about why diets suck. They're restrictive, joyless, and designed to fail. The cabbage soup diet? A fart-filled nightmare. Keto? Sure, if you love meat sweats and missing bread. Intermittent fasting? Congrats, you're just hungry and cranky all the time. The list goes on. Diets take away the simple joy of eating and replace it with spreadsheets, apps, and a constant sense of failure. Enough is enough.

This book isn't here to sell you another diet. It's here to help you flip the bird to all the bullshit rules and reclaim your right to enjoy food without shame. We're going to laugh at the absurdity of diet culture, embrace the beauty of food freedom, and, most importantly, learn how to stop giving a fuck about what anyone else thinks about your plate.

We're not chasing perfection here—because spoiler alert, it doesn't exist. We're not counting calories, tracking macros, or pretending that cauliflower pizza is the same as the real thing. (It's not. Let's stop lying to ourselves.) We're here to celebrate food, love our bodies, and live a life that's full, delicious, and completely free of guilt.

So buckle up. We're about to take a wild, hilarious, and sometimes messy ride through the world of food freedom. There will be swearing, there will be brutal honesty, and there will definitely be donuts. Let's send diet culture packing, one bite at a time.

Because life is too fucking short to eat bland chicken and cry over lettuce. Let's eat, laugh, and live our best damn lives. You ready? Let's do this.

Chapter 1

What the Fuck Is Diet Culture, and Why Is It Ruining Everything?

Food Guilt 101: How the World Convinced Us a Cookie Is a Moral Failing

Let's start with the obvious: food guilt is absolute bullshit. Somewhere along the line, society decided that eating wasn't just about survival or joy—it was about proving your moral superiority. The result? Every bite of food now comes with a side of judgment, shame, and a steaming pile of unnecessary guilt. And for what? A cookie? A slice of pizza? A f*cking bagel? It's time we take a closer look at how the hell we got here and why we need to kick this nonsense to the curb.

First, let's talk about the origins of food guilt. Back in the day—like, *way* back—eating was simple. You hunted, gathered, cooked, and ate, no calorie counting required. But fast-forward to the 20th century, and suddenly everything changed. Thanks to diet culture, the food on your plate became a reflection of your character. Eating a salad? You're disciplined and virtuous. Eating fries? You're a lazy slob with no self-control. This kind of thinking is not only absurd, but it's also dangerous.

Because newsflash: your worth has absolutely nothing to do with your lunch order.

Diet culture loves to assign morality to food. It divides everything into "good" and "bad," "clean" and "dirty," "allowed" and "forbidden." Carrots are good, but cake is bad. Quinoa is clean, but pasta is dirty. Kale is a saint, but bacon is the devil incarnate. And if you dare to eat something from the "bad" list? Boom—instant guilt, shame, and a free ticket to the self-loathing express. But here's the thing: food doesn't have morals. It's just food. A cookie isn't evil, and a salad doesn't make you a saint. The only thing they have in common is that they're both delicious.

Let's not forget how diet culture uses guilt as a marketing tool. Think about all the products out there labeled "guilt-free." Guilt-free ice cream. Guilt-free snacks. Guilt-free fucking chocolate bars. As if enjoying a treat is something you should feel guilty about in the first place. The message is clear: if you're eating something you actually enjoy, you're doing something wrong. It's manipulative as hell, and it's time we stop falling for it.

Now, let's get personal. Think about the last time you ate something "bad." Maybe it was a slice of cake at a birthday party, or a bag of chips while binge-watching Netflix. Did you enjoy it? Probably. Did you also spend the next hour beating yourself up over it? Definitely. That's food guilt in action, and it's a total buzzkill. It takes something that's supposed to bring you joy and turns it into a source of stress and self-hatred. And for what? A moment of pleasure? A little indulgence? It's not worth it.

Here's another fun fact: food guilt doesn't just ruin your mood—it can actually mess with your health. Studies show that feeling guilty about food can increase stress, which in turn can screw with your digestion, sleep, and overall well-being. So not only does food guilt make you feel like crap emotionally, but it also has physical consequences. Meanwhile, enjoying your food without guilt can do wonders for your body and mind. So next time you're tempted to feel bad about eating a cookie, remember: guilt is the real health hazard, not sugar.

Diet culture also loves to prey on our insecurities. It tells us that if we just eat the "right" foods and avoid the "wrong" ones, we'll be healthier, happier, and hotter. But the reality is much more complicated. Health isn't determined by a single meal or even a single diet—it's a combination of genetics, lifestyle, and a whole bunch of other factors that have nothing to do with whether or not you ate dessert last night. And happiness? That's not something you can achieve by cutting carbs or drinking green juice. In fact, it's probably the opposite.

Let's talk about one of diet culture's biggest lies: the idea that eating "bad" foods will ruin your progress. Whether you're trying to lose weight, build muscle, or just feel better in your own skin, diet culture wants you to believe that one donut can undo weeks of effort. But guess what? That's not how the human body works. Your progress isn't measured by a single meal—it's the result of consistent habits over time. So go ahead and eat the damn donut. It's not going to ruin anything, except maybe your ability to take diet culture seriously.

So how do we break free from food guilt? It starts with challenging the narratives we've been fed (pun intended) our entire lives. The next time you catch yourself feeling guilty about food, ask yourself: Where is this guilt coming from? Is it based on fact, or is it diet culture whispering lies in your ear? Chances are, it's the latter. Recognizing the source of your guilt is the first step in letting it go.

Another way to fight food guilt is to give yourself permission to eat what you love. No rules, no restrictions, no judgment. Just eat the foods that make you happy, and enjoy every bite. This might feel weird or even scary at first, especially if you've been stuck in the diet mindset for a long time. But the more you practice, the easier it gets. And the best part? The freedom and joy you'll feel when you finally stop judging yourself for eating a cookie.

Finally, remember this: food is not your enemy. It's not something to fear, avoid, or feel guilty about. It's fuel, nourishment, and—most importantly—pleasure. Eating is one of life's greatest joys, and you deserve to enjoy it without guilt or shame. So the next time diet culture tries to convince you that a cookie is a moral failing, tell it to f*ck off and enjoy your snack in peace.

Food guilt might be diet culture's greatest weapon, but it doesn't have to be yours. By challenging the lies, embracing food freedom, and giving yourself permission to enjoy eating, you can reclaim your relationship with food and live your life guilt-free. Because life is too short to waste on diet culture's bullsh*t—and way too short to skip dessert.

Let's dive into one of the biggest lies diet culture has ever sold us: the Skinny Fairy Tale. You know the one. It goes something like this: "Once upon a time, you were unhappy, unlovable, and unsatisfied with your life. But then you got thin, and everything magically fell into place. The end." Sounds nice, right? Too bad it's complete and utter bullsh*t. Thinness doesn't fix your life. It doesn't make you happier, healthier, or more successful. All it does is make you... well, thin. That's it. Let's unpack this garbage story and why it needs to die a fiery death.

First off, let's address the elephant in the room: thinness is not a universal key to happiness. Sure, diet culture loves to make it look that way with its before-and-after photos, its "transformation" stories, and its endless promises of a better life just waiting for you on the other side of weight loss. But here's the thing: thin people are just as likely to be unhappy as anyone else. They still have bills, breakups, bad hair days, and existential crises. Being thin doesn't shield you from the realities of life, and anyone who says otherwise is selling you snake oil.

Diet culture also loves to link thinness with success. It tells us that if we just lose the weight, we'll finally land the dream job, get the perfect partner, and become the confident, flawless versions of ourselves we've always wanted to be. But newsflash: confidence doesn't come from a number on the scale. It comes from how you feel about yourself, not what size jeans you wear. There are plenty of confident, badass people who don't fit the "thin" mold, and they're living proof that success has nothing to do with your waistline.

And let's not forget how diet culture uses fear to sell its Skinny Fairy Tale. It whispers, "If you don't lose the weight, you'll never be happy. You'll never find love. You'll never be enough." It preys on your insecurities and convinces you that thinness is the answer to all your problems. But here's the truth: the only thing that will make you happy is learning to love and accept yourself exactly as you are. Because no amount of weight loss will fill the void if you're not happy with yourself on the inside.

Now, let's talk about health. Diet culture loves to equate thinness with health, as if the two are interchangeable. But guess what? They're not. You can be thin and unhealthy, just like you can be not-so-thin and perfectly healthy. Health is about so much more than your weight—it's about your overall well-being, including your mental health, your relationships, and your quality of life. And let's be real: obsessing over your weight and denying yourself the foods you love isn't exactly the picture of health.

The Skinny Fairy Tale also ignores the fact that bodies come in all shapes and sizes. Some people are naturally thin, some are naturally curvy, and some fall somewhere in between. Trying to force your body into a shape it wasn't meant to be is like trying to squeeze into jeans that are two sizes too small—it's uncomfortable, unsustainable, and completely unnecessary. Your body is not a problem to be solved. It's your home, and it deserves to be loved and respected, no matter its size.

And let's not forget the double standard that diet culture loves to push. Thinness is celebrated, but how you get there doesn't seem to matter. Starving yourself? Skipping meals? Exercising to the point of exhaustion? Diet culture will applaud you for your "dedication" and "willpower," even if it's clearly wrecking your mental and physical health. Meanwhile, someone who's not thin but is living a balanced, happy, and healthy life is ignored or judged. It's f*cked up, and it needs to stop.

Let's also talk about the emotional toll of chasing the Skinny Fairy Tale. Dieting, restricting, and obsessing over your weight is exhausting. It drains your energy, your joy, and your self-esteem. And for what? So you can fit into a smaller size? So you can post a "transformation" photo on Instagram? It's not worth it. Life is too short to spend it hating your body and chasing an impossible ideal.

So how do we break free from the Skinny Fairy Tale? It starts with challenging the narratives we've been taught. The next time you catch yourself thinking, "If I just lose the weight, I'll be happy," ask yourself: Is that really true? What do I believe thinness will give me, and is there another way to achieve it? Chances are, the happiness, confidence, and self-worth you're seeking have nothing to do with your weight and everything to do with how you treat yourself.

Another way to fight back is to celebrate bodies of all shapes and sizes—not just thin ones. Surround yourself with images, stories, and role models who reflect the diversity of real bodies, not the narrow ideal that diet culture promotes. Follow body-positive influencers, read books that challenge diet culture, and remind yourself every day that your worth is not determined by your size.

Finally, remember that your body is not a project. It's not something to be fixed, improved, or transformed. It's a living, breathing, beautiful thing that carries you through life, and it deserves to be treated with love and respect. So instead of chasing the Skinny Fairy Tale, focus on building a life that brings you joy, fulfillment, and peace—regardless of your size.

Thinness doesn't fix sh*t. It doesn't make you a better person, a happier person, or a more successful person. But loving and accepting yourself exactly as you are? That's the real happily ever after. So let's ditch the fairy tale and start living our best lives, one unapologetic bite at a time.

Sneaky Diet Culture: How It's Infiltrating Your Instagram and Whispering Lies Into Your Ear

Let's talk about sneaky diet culture. It's like that shady ex who keeps showing up at your favorite bar, pretending to be "different" now, while still being the same manipulative asshole. Diet culture has rebranded itself, slapped on some yoga pants, and started calling itself "wellness." It's ditched the obvious slogans like "Lose 10 Pounds Fast!" and replaced them with sneaky little whispers like "Clean Eating," "Detox Your Body," and "Wellness Journey." And thanks to Instagram, it's infiltrated your life like a thief in the night, stealing your self-esteem one filtered photo at a time.

Let's start with the basics: what the fuck is diet culture doing on Instagram in the first place? It's dressed up as #inspiration, #motivation, and #fitspo, and it's everywhere. Your feed is flooded with influencers doing handstands on beaches, holding green smoothies like they're Oscars, and smiling through the pain of their "cleanse day." Their captions are filled with phrases like "treat your body like a temple" and "nothing tastes as good as healthy feels." Meanwhile, you're sitting there with a pizza slice, feeling like a failure for not living up to their kale-and-quinoa lifestyle. Spoiler: it's all bullshit.

Here's the truth: most of those influencers don't actually live the lives they're selling. They're taking 87 photos to get the perfect angle, editing out their cellulite, and hiding the fact that they just ate an entire box of cookies off-camera. But diet culture doesn't want you to know that. It wants you to believe that their perfect bodies and perfect lives are the result of their "clean eating" and "dedication." It's a scam, and you're the target.

Diet culture is sneaky as hell, and Instagram is its playground. Think about those "What I Eat in a Day" posts. They're designed to look relatable and inspiring, but they're actually just a guilt trap. The influencer shows you their tiny breakfast smoothie, their sad little salad for lunch, and their three almonds for a snack, and suddenly you're questioning why your meals don't look like that. But here's the thing: no one eats like that all the time—not even them. They're just not showing you the midnight binge or the reality of being hungry and miserable.

Then there are the "wellness" brands sliding into your feed like the worst kind of DMs. They're selling detox teas, skinny coffees, and magic powders that promise to make you lighter, healthier, and, let's be honest, more Instagram-worthy. These products are garbage. They don't do what they claim, and most of them are just overpriced laxatives wrapped in pretty packaging. But diet culture knows that if it slaps the word "wellness" on something, it can sell you anything—even a literal pile of crap.

Diet culture also loves to co-opt terms that should be empowering. "Intuitive eating"? Hijacked. "Self-care"? Twisted into a justification for diet restrictions. "Balance"? Now code for eating a salad so you can "earn" dessert. It's like diet culture is playing a game of telephone, taking perfectly good ideas and turning them into tools of guilt and shame.

And let's not forget the influencers who insist they're "not on a diet," but everything they post screams otherwise. They'll say things like, "I just love eating clean—it's not a diet, it's a lifestyle!" Meanwhile, their "lifestyle" is a full-time job of counting macros, avoiding carbs, and obsessing over their body fat percentage. But because they're not using the word "diet," they can pretend they're above it all. Newsflash: a diet by any other name is still a diet.

One of the sneakiest tricks diet culture uses on Instagram is the comparison game. You see someone's transformation photo, and suddenly you're comparing your body to theirs, wondering why you don't look like that. But here's the thing: transformation photos are bullshit. They're curated, filtered, and often staged. They don't show the full picture, like the hours of workouts, the calorie restrictions, and the mental toll of obsessing over every bite. Comparing yourself to those photos is like comparing a blooper reel to a highlight reel—it's not fair, and it's not real.

So how do you fight back against sneaky diet culture on Instagram? Step one: curate your feed like your mental health depends on it— because it does. Unfollow anyone who makes you feel like shit about yourself, no matter how many followers they have or how "inspiring" they claim to be. Instead, follow accounts that promote body positivity, food freedom, and realness. Look for people who show their stretch marks, eat burgers without apology, and call out diet culture for the garbage fire it is.

Step two: call out the bullsh*t when you see it. The next time you see a post promoting detox teas or "clean eating," don't just scroll past— challenge it. Comment, share, or just laugh at it with your friends. The more we collectively call out diet culture, the less power it has to fuck with us.

Step three: remind yourself that Instagram is not real life. It's a curated highlight reel, not a reflection of reality. Just because someone posts their green smoothie doesn't mean they didn't also eat a bag of chips.

And just because someone looks happy in a bikini doesn't mean they're happy in real life. Social media is full of smoke and mirrors, and the sooner you stop believing the illusion, the better off you'll be.

Step four: practice food freedom in your own life. Eat the pizza without guilt. Skip the gym if you're tired. Order dessert just because you feel like it. The more you embrace your own food freedom, the less power diet culture has over you. And the best part? You'll actually enjoy your life instead of living in constant fear of carbs.

Finally, remember this: diet culture may be sneaky, but you're smarter. You can see through the lies, the filters, and the marketing bullshit. You know that food isn't the enemy, your body isn't a problem to be solved, and Instagram doesn't define your worth. So the next time diet culture tries to whisper lies into your ear, tell it to fuck off—and then eat a donut for good measure.

Diet culture may be everywhere, but it doesn't have to control you. You've got the power to curate your feed, challenge the bullshit, and live your life on your terms. So go ahead, take back your Instagram, and let diet culture know it's no longer welcome. You deserve better—and you're too badass to settle for less.

Chapter 2

Fad Diets Are the Drunk Exes of the Food World

The Most WTF Diets We've Tried: From Eating Only Cabbage to Licking Air

Let's get one thing straight: fad diets are like the drunk ex you swear you're done with, but somehow, you keep going back for another round of misery. They're seductive as hell, promising you quick results, a better body, and maybe even eternal happiness, but they always end the same way—with you feeling like shit and wondering why you ever believed them in the first place. And let's be honest, some of these diets are so fucking absurd they sound like dares gone wrong.

Let's start with one of the classics: the *Cabbage Soup Diet*. This gem promises you'll lose weight fast by eating nothing but a bottomless pit of cabbage soup for a week. Sounds great, right? Until you realize that eating the same bland, fart-inducing sludge three times a day is a form of cruel and unusual punishment. Sure, you might lose a few pounds, but it's mostly water weight and the sheer will to live. And don't even think about being around other people—the side effects include enough gas to power a small city.

Then there's the *Grapefruit Diet*, which is basically a cult dedicated to worshiping the world's sourest fruit. The premise? Eat half a grapefruit before every meal, and the magical enzymes will melt your fat away. Spoiler alert: grapefruits aren't magical, and they sure as hell aren't going to turn your double chin into a jawline. All they do is make your mouth feel like it's been punched by citrus while you dream about real food.

Next up, we have the *Master Cleanse*, also known as the Lemonade Diet. Except this isn't your fun summer lemonade—it's a psychotic mix of lemon juice, cayenne pepper, and maple syrup that you're supposed to drink *instead* of eating. For ten days. TEN. FUCKING. DAYS. You're basically starving yourself while pretending that spicy lemonade is a meal. By day three, you're hallucinating cheeseburgers, and by day ten, you've lost weight, sure—but also your sanity, your dignity, and possibly your friends.

And let's not forget the *Air Diet*. Yes, you read that right. There are diets out there where people literally pretend to eat food but don't actually consume anything because "air is enough." I don't know who needs to hear this, but air is NOT FOOD. Unless you're a plant and can photosynthesize (spoiler: you can't), this is just a one-way ticket to starvation and a lifetime of therapy.

The *Hollywood Cookie Diet* is another fan favorite, especially if you've ever wished your meals could be replaced with glorified cardboard. The idea is to eat these "special" cookies for breakfast, lunch, and snacks, and then have a "sensible dinner." Sounds cute, right? Wrong. These cookies taste like a sad combination of sawdust and broken dreams, and after three days, you're ready to set fire to the whole box and eat an actual cookie for once.

Oh, and let's talk about *Juice Cleanses*. These are like the Instagram influencers of diets—pretty to look at, but useless in real life. The concept is simple: drink nothing but cold-pressed juice for days or weeks on end to "detox" your body. Except, fun fact, your liver and kidneys already detox your body just fine. All a juice cleanse does is leave you hangry, lightheaded, and broke because, let's face it, that shit is expensive.

The *Tapeworm Diet* deserves a special mention for being both horrifying and batshit insane. Yes, this was a thing people actually did. The idea? Swallow a pill containing a live tapeworm, let it live in your intestines and "eat your calories," and then somehow remove it later. Besides being disgusting, it's also wildly unsafe. You might lose weight, sure, but you're also risking death, and honestly, I'd rather just eat the damn cake.

Then there's the *Raw Food Diet*, which is fine if you love the idea of living like a rabbit. Everything you eat has to be raw, unprocessed, and, of course, cold as hell. No cooking, no frying, no baking—just raw fruits, veggies, and whatever else you can stomach. The only good thing about this diet is that you don't have to do dishes, but even that isn't worth the price of eating cold zucchini noodles while your friends are enjoying pizza.

Let's not overlook the *Baby Food Diet*, which involves eating tiny jars of mush designed for literal babies. Why? Because portion control, apparently. Sure, it's low-calorie, but it's also low on flavor, satisfaction, and anything remotely resembling an adult meal. You're essentially regressing to infancy, all while pretending you're a sophisticated health guru.

And last but not least, we have *Keto*. Now, keto isn't as batshit crazy as some of the others on this list, but it still has its moments. Sure, the idea of eating bacon and cheese sounds great at first, but after a week without bread, you start contemplating crimes just to get your hands on a bagel. Plus, there's the infamous "keto flu," where your body rebels against the lack of carbs and leaves you feeling like death warmed over. Fun times.

The problem with all these diets—besides the fact that they're ridiculous—is that they're unsustainable. You can't live on cabbage soup, grapefruit, or spicy lemonade forever. Eventually, you'll go back to eating normal food, and guess what? The weight you lost comes right back, along with a healthy dose of shame and frustration. It's a vicious cycle, and it's exactly what diet culture wants.

So what's the alternative? Simple: stop dieting. Stop chasing quick fixes and start focusing on building a relationship with food that doesn't involve misery and self-loathing. Eat what you love, listen to your body, and for the love of all that's holy, stop swallowing tapeworm pills.

Fad diets are nothing more than drunk exes—fun for a hot second, but ultimately toxic, manipulative, and not worth your time. Kick them to the curb, block their number, and move on with your life. Because you deserve better, and your relationship with food deserves better too.

The Quick Fix Fantasy: Why Your "Summer Body" Dreams Always End in Snacks

Let's talk about the fantasy that keeps diet culture alive and kicking: the idea that there's a magical, easy, quick fix that will transform you into the bronzed, shredded, beach goddess (or god) you've always dreamed of being. You know the one—where you lose 20 pounds in a month, wake up with abs, and finally get to post thirst traps without wondering if anyone's judging your cellulite. It's the pipe dream that sells detox teas, waist trainers, and every other scam product under the sun. And it's also the biggest crock of shit you'll ever buy into.

Here's the cold, hard truth: quick fixes don't work. They never have, and they never will. Sure, they might give you temporary results, but they're also guaranteed to leave you miserable, starving, and plotting a violent overthrow of the kale industry. And worst of all? The weight you lose always comes back, dragging along a few extra pounds for good measure—like a toxic ex who just won't let go.

Let's break down why the quick fix fantasy is such a seductive pile of bullshit. First, it promises speed. Diet culture knows we're impatient as hell, so it dangles phrases like "Lose 10 pounds in 10 days!" and "Drop a dress size overnight!" in front of us like candy. And because we're human, we fall for it. Who wouldn't want instant results without the hassle of long-term effort? It's like signing up for a gym membership and expecting to wake up the next day looking like a Greek statue. Spoiler: that's not how bodies work.

Next, there's the illusion of effortlessness. Quick fixes love to pretend they're easy. "Just drink this magical shake twice a day!" "Pop this pill before meals, and watch the fat melt away!" "Wear this waist trainer, and your abs will practically carve themselves!" It's all designed to make you believe you can transform your body without lifting a finger. But here's the thing: anything worth having takes effort, and that includes a healthy relationship with food and your body. There's no such thing as effortless weight loss, and anyone who says otherwise is lying—or trying to sell you something.

And let's not forget the most dangerous part of the quick fix fantasy: the promise of perfection. Every ad, every influencer, every before-and-after photo screams the same message: "If you just do this one thing, your life will be perfect." You'll be thin, confident, happy, successful, and loved. But here's the truth: losing weight doesn't magically solve all your problems. It doesn't pay your bills, fix your relationships, or make your boss less of an asshole. It just makes you... thinner. And if you're not happy with yourself at the start, you're sure as hell not going to be happy at the finish line.

So why do these quick fixes always end in snacks? Because they're unsustainable as fuck. You can only drink lemon-cayenne-maple syrup water for so long before your body rebels and demands a cheeseburger. You can only eat 1,000 calories a day before you find yourself elbow-deep in a bag of chips at 2 a.m., cursing the diet gods. Quick fixes rely on restriction, and restriction always leads to rebellion. It's basic psychology: tell yourself you can't have something, and suddenly it's all you can think about.

Let's get personal. Think about the last time you tried a quick fix. Maybe it was a juice cleanse, a low-carb diet, or some other miserable scheme. At first, it felt great. You were motivated, you saw results, and you thought, "This is it! I've finally cracked the code!" But then reality set in. You got hungry. You got tired. You got fed up. And before you knew it, you were bingeing on everything you'd been denying yourself, feeling like a failure and swearing to "start over" on Monday. Sound familiar? That's the quick fix cycle, and it's a soul-sucking merry-go-round you deserve to get off.

Quick fixes also set you up for failure by turning food into the enemy. They make you afraid of carbs, sugar, fat, and pretty much anything that tastes good. They convince you that eating "bad" foods will ruin your progress and make you unworthy of love and happiness. But here's the truth: food isn't the enemy. It's not something to be feared, avoided, or demonized. It's fuel, pleasure, and a fundamental part of life. And anyone who tells you otherwise is full of shit.

Let's not ignore the emotional toll of quick fixes, either. They fuck with your head in the worst way possible. Every time you "fail" at a quick fix, you feel like it's your fault. Like you're weak, undisciplined, and incapable of achieving your goals. But guess what? The problem isn't you—it's the diet. Quick fixes are designed to fail because they're based on unrealistic expectations and unsustainable practices. You're not failing the diet; the diet is failing you.

So how do we break free from the quick fix fantasy? First, we need to stop looking for shortcuts. There's no magic pill, no one-size-fits-all solution, and no overnight transformation. True health and happiness come from building sustainable habits, not chasing temporary results. It's not sexy, and it's definitely not fast, but it's the only thing that actually works.

Next, we need to challenge the narratives diet culture has fed us. The next time you see an ad promising rapid weight loss, ask yourself: "Is this realistic? Is this healthy? Is this something I can maintain for the rest of my life?" If the answer is no—and it usually is—walk away. Your time, energy, and mental health are worth more than falling for another scam.

We also need to redefine what success looks like. Instead of measuring your worth by the number on the scale or the size of your jeans, focus on how you feel. Are you energized? Are you enjoying your meals? Are you treating your body with kindness and respect? Those are the things that truly matter—not some arbitrary "summer body" goal that's as fleeting as a Snapchat story.

Finally, we need to embrace the fact that life is messy, imperfect, and delicious. Sometimes you're going to eat kale, and sometimes you're going to eat cake. Sometimes you'll hit the gym, and sometimes you'll binge-watch Netflix with a pint of ice cream. And that's okay. Balance isn't about being perfect—it's about making choices that nourish your body and soul, without guilt or shame.

The quick fix fantasy is just that—a fantasy. It's a shiny, seductive lie designed to keep you chasing something that doesn't exist. But you're smarter than that. You know that real change takes time, effort, and a whole lot of self-compassion. So ditch the detoxes, burn the waist trainers, and eat the fucking snacks. Your "summer body" is the one you already have, and it's worth celebrating just as it is.

Cleanse Culture: Why Your Liver Doesn't Need a Green Juice—Trust Me, It's Fine

Let's talk about cleanse culture, the most overpriced, overhyped bullshit diet culture has ever shoved down our throats—literally. It's the belief that your body is somehow "toxic" and desperately needs a detox to function. And who's swooping in to save the day? Juice cleanses, detox teas, and every snake oil salesman with a blender and a thirst for your money. They claim to "flush out toxins," "reset your system," and "boost your energy," all while charging you $12 a bottle for cold-pressed celery water. But here's the truth: your liver and kidneys already have this detox thing covered, and they're doing just fine without a goddamn green juice.

Cleanse culture operates on one big, fat lie: the idea that your body is dirty. It tells you that all those burgers, pizzas, and margaritas you've been enjoying are "toxic," and the only way to redeem yourself is to embark on a weeklong juice cleanse. Spoiler alert: your body is not a clogged sink, and you don't need a juice plumber to fix it. Your liver is a badass detox machine, working 24/7 to keep you alive and thriving. It doesn't need a green juice assist, and it definitely doesn't need you starving yourself in the name of wellness.

Let's break down what a juice cleanse actually is: expensive starvation. That's it. You're paying a ridiculous amount of money to drink liquefied kale and apple juice while denying your body the nutrients it actually needs. And for what? A little water weight loss? A false sense of purity? The chance to post a smug Instagram story about your "cleanse journey"? It's all smoke and mirrors, and the only thing getting cleansed is your bank account.

And can we talk about how disgusting these juices are? Sure, they look pretty in their little glass bottles with their pastel labels and minimalist fonts, but one sip and you realize you've just paid $15 to drink liquid lawn clippings. They try to disguise the misery with names like "Revitalize," "Glow," and "Green Goddess," but let's be real—they all taste like wet grass mixed with regret. And the ones that claim to be "sweet" just taste like someone whispered the word "pineapple" over a bucket of swamp water.

Now, let's get into the science—or lack thereof. Cleanse culture loves to throw around the word "toxins" without ever specifying what these so-called toxins actually are. It's just a vague, scary buzzword designed to make you panic and whip out your credit card. The truth is, if you have a functioning liver and kidneys, your body is already detoxing itself like a goddamn pro. Those organs don't need your overpriced juice—they need you to stop believing diet culture's lies.

And let's not forget the side effects of juice cleanses, which cleanse culture conveniently glosses over. You're constantly hungry, cranky as hell, and running to the bathroom every 15 minutes because your body is screaming, "What the fuck are you doing to me?!" Your energy levels plummet, your mood tanks, and by day three, you're fantasizing about eating solid food like it's a long-lost lover. But hey, at least you've "reset your system," right?

Cleanse culture also loves to slap the word "reset" on everything, as if your body is some kind of malfunctioning computer that just needs a hard reboot. But here's the thing: your body isn't a machine. It's a complex, self-regulating, miraculous organism that doesn't need you to micromanage it with carrot juice and wheatgrass shots. If you're feeling sluggish or bloated, the answer isn't a cleanse—it's probably just drinking more water, getting enough sleep, and maybe not eating an entire pizza in one sitting (but hey, no judgment if you do).

And let's not ignore the psychological damage cleanse culture does. It feeds into the idea that eating is something you need to "repent" for, as if enjoying a slice of cake or a bag of chips is a mortal sin. It turns food into a moral issue and convinces you that deprivation is a form of virtue. But here's the truth: eating is not something you need to atone for, and starvation is not a fucking virtue. You're allowed to enjoy your food without feeling the need to "cleanse" yourself afterward.

Then there are the celebrity endorsements, which are the cherry on top of this bullshit sundae. Every time a Kardashian or some random influencer promotes a detox tea or juice cleanse, you can bet they're not actually drinking that shit. They're just cashing a fat check while you're choking down spinach juice and pretending it's delicious. Meanwhile, they're probably eating caviar and laughing all the way to the bank.

So why does cleanse culture keep thriving? Because it preys on our insecurities. It tells us we're not good enough, not pure enough, not healthy enough, and then offers us a quick, easy fix to solve all our problems. It's diet culture at its sneakiest and most manipulative, and it's time we call it out for the scam it is.

So how do we break free from cleanse culture? First, stop believing the hype. The next time someone tries to sell you a detox product, ask yourself: What toxins is this supposed to remove? How does it work? Where's the evidence? Chances are, there are no answers—just vague promises and clever marketing.

Second, trust your body. Your liver, kidneys, and digestive system are already doing the detox work for you, and they're doing it better than any green juice ever could. If you want to support your body, focus on eating a balanced diet, staying hydrated, and giving it the rest it needs—not starving it in the name of a cleanse.

Third, give yourself permission to enjoy food without guilt. Food is not toxic. It's not something you need to "cleanse" yourself of. It's nourishment, pleasure, and a fundamental part of life. Eat the burger, drink the wine, and enjoy the damn cupcake. Your body can handle it.

Finally, spread the word. The more we call out cleanse culture for the scam it is, the less power it has to manipulate us. Share this truth with your friends, laugh at the absurdity of it all, and remind yourself that you're smarter than diet culture's bullshit.

25

Cleanse culture is nothing more than overpriced misery wrapped in a shiny package. Your liver doesn't need a green juice, your system doesn't need a reset, and your worth is not determined by how "clean" your eating is. So the next time someone tries to sell you a cleanse, tell them to fuck off—and then go enjoy some solid food like the badass you are.

Chapter 3

Food Isn't the Villain —Your Brain Is

Carbs Aren't Satan's Spawn: Stop Acting Like a Bagel Is a Personal Attack

Let's talk about carbs—the most demonized, misunderstood, and unfairly targeted food group of all time. Diet culture has spent decades convincing us that carbs are the enemy, turning everything from bread to pasta into public enemies number one and two. But here's the real tea: carbs are not out to get you. They're not lurking in the shadows, waiting to sabotage your health and happiness. They're just food, for fuck's sake. It's your brain—and diet culture whispering lies into it— that's making you act like a bagel is a goddamn supervillain.

First, let's clear something up: carbs are not inherently bad. In fact, they're kind of essential. Your body literally *needs* carbohydrates to function. They're your primary source of energy, the fuel that keeps you moving, thinking, and breathing. Cutting them out entirely is like trying to run a car without gas—it's not going to end well. And yet, diet culture has managed to turn carbs into the nutritional equivalent of Voldemort, convincing us that even looking at a slice of bread will send us straight to dietary hell.

Let's take a little stroll down memory lane to the birth of the anti-carb hysteria. It all started with the Atkins diet, which declared war on carbs in the late '90s and early 2000s. Suddenly, bread, pasta, and potatoes were the villains of every weight-loss story, and protein was hailed as the hero. Then came keto, which took the anti-carb agenda to a whole new level, demanding that you eat so few carbs your body starts eating its own fat for fuel. Sure, you might lose weight, but you'll also lose your sanity—and any joy you once had for food.

But why, exactly, are carbs so demonized? Because they're easy to scapegoat. They're comforting, delicious, and often associated with indulgence, which makes them an easy target for diet culture's shame machine. Plus, cutting carbs can lead to quick water weight loss, which diet culture loves to parade around as "proof" that carbs are bad. What they don't tell you is that this weight comes right back as soon as you eat a bagel—and no, it's not because carbs are evil. It's because your body needs them, and it's holding onto every crumb like a kid who's been grounded from candy.

Here's the thing about carbs: they're fucking awesome. Bread is basically a hug in food form. Pasta is a work of art. Potatoes? Those glorious bastards can be mashed, fried, baked, and roasted, and they're delicious every single way. Carbs are the backbone of comfort food, the MVPs of any meal, and the lifeblood of hangover cures everywhere. Demonizing them is like trying to cancel puppies or sunsets—it just doesn't make sense.

Now, let's talk about the mental gymnastics diet culture makes you do to avoid carbs. Suddenly, you're spiraling over the bread basket at dinner, debating whether one slice will ruin your progress. You're Googling "low-carb alternatives" and ending up with cauliflower everything—rice, pizza crust, even goddamn gnocchi. Look, I love cauliflower as much as the next person, but it's not rice. It's not pizza. It's a vegetable, and it deserves better than being forced into roles it was never meant to play.

And don't even get me started on the guilt. Diet culture has weaponized carbs, turning every bite of bread or bowl of pasta into a moral failing. You eat a donut, and suddenly you're spiraling, thinking, "Why did I do that? I'm so weak. I'll never reach my goals." But guess what? Eating a donut doesn't make you weak—it makes you human. Food is not a test of willpower, and you're not a bad person for enjoying it.

Let's also address the double standard that comes with carb shaming. On one hand, you're told to avoid carbs at all costs because they're "bad" for you. On the other hand, you're bombarded with images of influencers eating avocado toast and croissants on Instagram, looking impossibly chic and carefree. The message is clear: carbs are only okay if you're thin enough to "deserve" them. Fuck that noise. Carbs are for everyone, no matter what size jeans you wear.

The real villain here isn't carbs—it's diet culture and the lies it feeds your brain. It's the voice that tells you carbs are the reason you're not happy, healthy, or confident. It's the voice that makes you feel guilty for eating a slice of cake at a party or grabbing a bagel on your way to work. It's the voice that keeps you stuck in a cycle of restriction, bingeing, and shame. And it's time to tell that voice to shut the fuck up.

So how do we break free from carb guilt? First, start questioning the bullshit. The next time someone tells you carbs are bad, ask them why. Chances are, they won't have a solid answer—just a bunch of regurgitated diet culture talking points. Remind yourself that carbs are a normal, healthy part of a balanced diet, and that your body needs them to function.

Second, stop labeling foods as "good" or "bad." Carbs aren't evil, just like kale isn't holy. They're both food, and they both have a place in your life. It's all about balance, not perfection. Some days you'll eat quinoa, and some days you'll eat cake. Both are valid choices, and neither one defines your worth.

Third, start listening to your body instead of diet culture. If you're craving carbs, eat them. Don't try to suppress the craving with bullshit substitutes or deny yourself until you end up bingeing. Honor your hunger, honor your cravings, and trust that your body knows what it needs.

Finally, start celebrating carbs for the glorious, delicious, life-giving heroes they are. Eat the bread. Enjoy the pasta. Savor the pizza. Carbs aren't out to ruin your life—they're here to make it better. And you deserve to enjoy them without guilt, shame, or second-guessing.

Carbs aren't Satan's spawn. They're not the reason for your problems, and they're not out to destroy you. They're food, plain and simple. And it's time we stop acting like a bagel is a personal attack and start treating carbs with the love and respect they deserve. So go ahead— toast that bread, twirl that spaghetti, and let carbs back into your life. Your brain might freak out at first, but trust me, it'll thank you later.

Your Hunger Is Not a F*cking Character Flaw: Trust Your Body—It Knows What It's Doing

Let's get one thing straight: hunger is not the enemy. It's not a moral failing, a sign of weakness, or a personal shortcoming. Hunger is your body's way of saying, "Hey, I need some fuel to keep this show running." But diet culture, in all its manipulative glory, has convinced us that feeling hungry is something to be ashamed of. That if you're hungry, you're doing something wrong. Well, that's a steaming pile of horseshit, and it's time to set the record straight.

First of all, let's address the absurdity of demonizing hunger. Hunger is literally one of the most basic, natural, and necessary biological signals your body sends you. It's right up there with breathing, blinking, and needing to pee. Ignoring your hunger is like ignoring your bladder screaming for relief—you can try to tough it out, but eventually, it's going to end in disaster. And yet, diet culture has made us believe that suppressing hunger is some kind of badge of honor. Newsflash: it's not. It's just stupid.

Diet culture has a whole arsenal of tricks to make you feel guilty for being hungry. It tells you that you should be able to "control" your hunger, like it's some unruly toddler throwing a tantrum in the grocery store. It glorifies phrases like "appetite suppressant" and "stay strong," as if resisting a snack is the moral equivalent of saving a puppy from a burning building. And don't even get me started on the "hunger hacks" designed to trick your body into thinking it's not hungry. Eating ice cubes? Drinking gallons of water? Sniffing peppermint oil? What the actual fuck?

Let me tell you something: hunger is not something to hack, suppress, or outsmart. It's something to honor. Your body is not a malfunctioning machine that needs to be tricked into silence—it's a highly intelligent system that knows what it needs. Ignoring your hunger is like ignoring your car's gas light and expecting it to keep running on empty. Sure, you might get a few more miles, but eventually, you're going to break down.

And let's talk about the shame that comes with feeling hungry. Diet culture has us convinced that hunger is a sign of failure. That if you're hungry, you're greedy, indulgent, or lacking in willpower. But guess what? Hunger is not a character flaw—it's a survival mechanism. Your body is designed to keep you alive, and hunger is its way of making sure you don't starve to death. Feeling hungry doesn't make you weak; it makes you human.

Now, let's get into the science of hunger, because facts are the ultimate diet culture destroyer. Hunger is regulated by a complex system of hormones, including ghrelin (the hunger hormone) and leptin (the fullness hormone). When your body needs fuel, ghrelin levels rise, sending a signal to your brain that it's time to eat. When you've had enough, leptin steps in to let you know you're full. It's a beautifully orchestrated system that's been keeping humans alive for thousands of years—long before calorie counting apps and juice cleanses were a thing.

But diet culture loves to mess with this system. Restrictive diets, fasting, and constant calorie deficits throw your hunger hormones out of whack, making it harder for your body to regulate itself. That's why dieting often leads to bingeing—your body is just trying to make up for the energy deficit you've been forcing it into. It's not a lack of willpower; it's biology.

So how do you start trusting your hunger? First, you need to unlearn the bullshit diet culture has taught you. The next time you feel hungry, instead of trying to suppress it or distract yourself, try listening to it. Ask yourself, "What does my body need right now?" Maybe it's a snack, maybe it's a meal, maybe it's a combination of carbs, protein, and fat. Whatever it is, honor it. Your body knows what it's doing, and it's time you started trusting it.

Second, stop labeling hunger as "good" or "bad." Hunger is not a moral issue—it's a physical one. Feeling hungry doesn't make you a bad person, just like feeling full doesn't make you a good person. They're just states of being, and both are completely normal. Stop judging yourself for your body's natural signals and start responding to them with compassion.

Third, start paying attention to your hunger cues. Diet culture has trained us to ignore these signals, but they're still there, waiting to be heard. Take a moment to check in with your body before, during, and after meals. Are you feeling satisfied? Energized? Still hungry? These cues are your body's way of guiding you, and the more you listen to them, the better you'll get at understanding what your body needs.

And let's not forget the importance of satisfaction. Diet culture loves to push the idea that eating is just about fuel, but that's a load of crap. Food is about more than just calories—it's about pleasure, connection, and joy. If you're eating a meal that doesn't satisfy you, you're going to keep feeling hungry, no matter how many calories you consume. So go ahead and eat the foods that make you happy, and don't let diet culture guilt you into thinking you should settle for bland chicken and steamed broccoli.

One of the biggest ways to rebuild trust with your hunger is to let go of food rules. Diet culture loves to impose rules like "don't eat after 7 p.m." or "only snack on veggies," but these rules are arbitrary and harmful. Your hunger doesn't operate on a schedule, and it doesn't care about diet culture's opinions. If you're hungry, eat. If you're not, don't. It's that simple.

Finally, remember that hunger is not your enemy—it's your ally. It's your body's way of keeping you alive, energized, and ready to take on the world. Instead of fighting it, try embracing it. Trust that your body knows what it's doing, and give it the fuel it needs to thrive.

Your hunger is not a fucking character flaw. It's not a sign of weakness or failure. It's a natural, beautiful, and essential part of being human. So stop treating it like an inconvenience, and start treating it like the vital signal it is. Honor your hunger, trust your body, and tell diet culture to fuck off. You've got this.

Eating Should Be Fun: Yes, That Means Pizza at Midnight Without the Side of Shame

Let's get one thing straight: eating is supposed to be enjoyable. It's one of life's simplest and greatest pleasures. Food is meant to be savored, celebrated, and shared—not agonized over, counted, or weighed like some kind of moral currency. And yet, diet culture has managed to suck all the joy out of eating, turning it into a battleground of guilt, shame, and anxiety. Well, fuck that noise. It's time to reclaim the fun in food, because life is too short to cry over a slice of pizza at midnight.

First of all, let's talk about the absurdity of food guilt. Somewhere along the line, we started acting like eating "fun" foods—pizza, burgers, ice cream—is some kind of moral failing. As if enjoying a plate of nachos automatically makes you a lazy, irresponsible slob. But guess what? It doesn't. Eating food you love doesn't make you a bad person; it makes you a person. Full stop.

Diet culture loves to divide food into two categories: "good" and "bad." Kale? Good. Donuts? Bad. Grilled chicken? Good. Fried chicken? Bad. It's like some twisted version of The Hunger Games where only "clean eaters" get to win. But here's the truth: food doesn't have morals. It's not good or bad—it's just food. And you're allowed to enjoy all of it without feeling like you need to go to confession afterward.

Let's not forget the ridiculous rules diet culture imposes on when and how we're allowed to eat. "No carbs after 6 p.m." "No snacks after dinner." "Only eat dessert on special occasions." Who the fuck came up with this nonsense? If you're hungry at midnight and pizza sounds like the answer to your prayers, then guess what? Pizza is the answer to your prayers. You don't need permission from some arbitrary set of rules to eat what you want, when you want it.

And can we talk about the joy of late-night eating? There's something magical about biting into a slice of pizza at midnight, when the world is quiet and you're wrapped in the warm, cheesy embrace of carbs. Or sneaking a spoonful of ice cream straight from the carton while binge-watching your favorite show. These moments are not crimes—they're rituals. Little acts of rebellion against the joyless rules of diet culture.

Of course, diet culture loves to ruin everything by slapping a side of shame onto these moments. You eat a slice of cake at a birthday party, and suddenly that little voice in your head is screaming, "You shouldn't have done that! Now you'll have to skip breakfast tomorrow!" But here's the thing: food is not a crime scene, and you don't need to punish yourself for eating it. You're allowed to enjoy a slice of cake without it turning into a goddamn courtroom drama.

Eating for pleasure is not only okay—it's necessary. Studies show that when you enjoy your food, you're more likely to feel satisfied and less likely to overeat. Pleasure is an essential part of the eating experience, and denying yourself that pleasure only leads to frustration, obsession, and, let's be real, eventual bingeing. So go ahead and eat the brownie. Savor every bite. It's not just okay—it's good for you.

One of the biggest lies diet culture tells us is that food should only be about fuel. "Food is just energy," they say. "You eat to live, not live to eat." Fuck that. Food is so much more than fuel. It's culture, connection, tradition, and joy. It's Sunday brunch with your best friends, Thanksgiving dinner with your family, and that perfect slice of cake on your birthday. Reducing food to a mere calorie count is like reducing music to sound waves—it misses the entire point.

Let's also address the idea that fun foods are somehow less "worthy" than their boring, "healthy" counterparts. Diet culture loves to glamorize bland, flavorless meals like grilled chicken and steamed broccoli, while demonizing pizza, pasta, and fried anything. But here's the truth: all food is worthy. Whether it's a kale salad or a bucket of fried chicken, it all has value—and so do you, no matter what you're eating.

And let's not ignore the social aspect of eating. Food is meant to be shared and enjoyed with others. But diet culture has turned it into a solitary, guilt-ridden act where you measure every bite and calculate every calorie. It's time to bring the fun back into food by embracing the joy of eating with friends and family. Order the appetizers. Share the dessert. Laugh, eat, and be merry. That's what food is all about.

So how do we start making eating fun again? First, throw out the fucking rulebook. The next time diet culture tells you not to eat carbs after dark or skip dessert, tell it to fuck off. You don't need rules to enjoy food—you just need permission from yourself.

Second, start listening to your body instead of the noise. What are you craving? What sounds good? What will make you feel happy and satisfied? Trust your instincts—they're smarter than you think.

Third, stop labeling foods as "good" or "bad." Instead, focus on what feels good for you. Some days that might be a green smoothie, and other days it might be a bacon cheeseburger. Both are valid choices, and neither one defines your worth.

Fourth, embrace the joy of eating with others. Share a meal, try new foods, and make memories. Food is about connection, and the best meals are the ones enjoyed with people you love.

Finally, let go of the guilt. Eating should be fun, not a chore or a source of stress. You're allowed to enjoy your food without overanalyzing every bite. So the next time you find yourself craving pizza at midnight, eat the fucking pizza. Savor it, enjoy it, and move on with your life.

Eating is one of life's greatest pleasures, and it's time we started treating it that way. Say goodbye to food guilt, throw caution to the wind, and embrace the delicious, messy, joyful experience of eating. Because life is too short to spend it crying over carbs and calculating calories. Eat the pizza, enjoy the dessert, and live your best fucking life.

Chapter 4

Smash the Scale Like It Owes You Money

The Scale Is a Lying Asshole: Why Your Self-Worth Has Nothing to Do With a Number

Let's talk about the scale—arguably the most manipulative, lying little asshole in your bathroom. It's the ultimate gaslighter, convincing you that your entire worth as a human being boils down to one number that changes depending on the time of day, how much water you drank, or whether you dared to eat a goddamn sandwich. It's time we stop giving this sneaky piece of metal so much fucking power and start seeing it for what it really is: a tool, not a judge, jury, or executioner.

First, let's break down the sheer absurdity of the scale's control over our lives. You step on it in the morning, hoping for validation, and if the number goes down, you feel like a fucking rockstar. But if it goes up— even by half a pound—you spiral into a pit of self-loathing and start Googling "how to lose weight overnight." Does that sound healthy? Does that sound normal? Hell no. It sounds like you're giving a $20 bathroom accessory the emotional power of a toxic ex.

Here's the truth: the number on the scale doesn't mean jack shit. It doesn't measure your health, your happiness, your kindness, your intelligence, or any of the things that actually matter. All it does is tell you how much gravity is currently pulling on your body—and guess what? Gravity fluctuates. You drink a glass of water? The scale goes up. You take a piss? The scale goes down. It's not rocket science; it's basic biology.

Diet culture, of course, loves to make the scale the star of the show. It pushes the idea that your weight is the ultimate marker of your success, your attractiveness, and your self-worth. It tells you that if the number on the scale isn't going down, you're failing. But here's a fun fact: diet culture is a lying sack of shit. Weight is just one small piece of the puzzle when it comes to health, and it's not even the most important one.

Let's not ignore the emotional abuse the scale dishes out on the daily. You wake up feeling good, proud of yourself for sticking to your goals, and then you step on the scale and BAM—it shits all over your mood. Suddenly, you're questioning everything. Did you eat too much yesterday? Should you skip breakfast today? What the fuck are you even doing with your life? All because of a number that's about as reliable as a Magic 8-Ball.

And can we talk about the ridiculous rituals we perform around the scale? You weigh yourself naked, after you pee, before you eat or drink anything, because heaven forbid the scale reflects the true reality of your body. You hold your breath, cross your fingers, and pray to the diet gods for a number that won't ruin your day. It's exhausting, it's degrading, and it's completely unnecessary.

Here's another mind-blowing truth: your weight can fluctuate by several pounds in a single day, and it has nothing to do with fat gain or loss. It's just water retention, food in your stomach, or hormonal shifts. But diet culture conveniently forgets to tell you that, because it wants you to obsess over every little change like it's the end of the world. Spoiler alert: it's not.

The scale also fails to account for all the amazing things your body does that have nothing to do with weight. It doesn't measure your strength, your endurance, your ability to hug your loved ones, or the fact that your legs carry you through life every damn day. Your body is so much more than a number, and it's time we started treating it that way.

So how do we break free from the scale's toxic grip? First, stop weighing yourself. Seriously, just stop. Put the scale in the closet, throw it in the dumpster, or smash it with a sledgehammer if you're feeling dramatic. The less you step on that lying asshole, the less power it has over you.

Second, start focusing on non-scale victories. Instead of measuring your success by your weight, measure it by how you feel, how strong you're getting, or how much energy you have. Celebrate the things that actually matter, like being able to run up the stairs without getting winded or finally nailing that yoga pose you've been working on.

Third, remind yourself that health is not a number. It's a combination of physical, mental, and emotional well-being, and it looks different for everyone. Your worth is not determined by your weight, and your health is not defined by the scale.

Fourth, start talking to yourself the way you would talk to a friend. If your bestie called you crying because the scale went up by two pounds, would you tell her she's a failure? Hell no. You'd remind her that weight fluctuates, that she's doing her best, and that she's a badass regardless of what the scale says. So why not extend that same kindness to yourself?

Finally, start living your life without letting the scale dictate your happiness. Eat the food you love, move your body in ways that feel good, and stop obsessing over a number that doesn't define you. Life is too short to spend it crying over the scale, and you deserve better.

The scale is a lying asshole, but it doesn't have to control you. You're so much more than a number, and it's time to start living like it. Smash the scale, take back your power, and start measuring your worth by the things that actually matter—like how much joy you bring to the world, how many laughs you share with your friends, and how fucking awesome you are. Because let's face it: you're pretty fucking awesome.

Breaking Up with Your Daily Weigh-In: It's Not You, It's the Scale

Let's face it: your relationship with the scale has been toxic for far too long. It's time for a breakup, and not one of those "let's still be friends" deals. This needs to be a full-blown, cold-turkey, block-its-number-and-delete-it-from-your-life kind of split. Why? Because the scale is the ultimate gaslighter, a manipulative little bastard that has you hanging onto every digit like your entire self-worth depends on it. Spoiler alert: it doesn't. It's time to kick that lying asshole to the curb and take back your sanity.

First, let's acknowledge how the scale has fucked with your head. You wake up, feeling good about yourself, ready to conquer the day. Then you step on the scale, and BAM—it shits all over your confidence. The number is higher than you expected, and suddenly your mood is in the gutter. You're questioning everything you ate yesterday, feeling guilty about that dessert you enjoyed, and plotting out a day of "compensatory" behavior, like skipping breakfast or doing an extra workout. Sound familiar? That's not a healthy relationship—that's emotional abuse.

And let's not pretend the scale is even accurate. It fluctuates more than your ex's excuses for why they couldn't text you back. You step on it in the morning, and it gives you one number. Step on it again after breakfast, and it's a whole other story. Drink a glass of water, and suddenly you're "heavier." Eat a meal, and it's like you've gained five pounds overnight. The scale doesn't care about your mental health—it just spits out numbers with zero context, leaving you to interpret them like some kind of twisted fortune teller.

The scale doesn't measure anything that actually matters. It doesn't tell you how strong you're getting, how much energy you have, or how badass you are for showing up for yourself every day. It doesn't measure your worth as a friend, a partner, or a human being. All it does is reflect your relationship with gravity at a specific moment in time— and guess what? That's not a measure of success, happiness, or health.

Breaking up with your daily weigh-in starts with understanding why you've been so attached to it in the first place. Diet culture has drilled into us that weight is the ultimate metric of health and success. That if the number is going down, we're winning, and if it's going up, we're failing. But here's the thing: weight is just one piece of a much larger puzzle, and it's not even the most important one. Your health, happiness, and overall well-being cannot and should not be reduced to a single number.

Let's also acknowledge the emotional rollercoaster the scale puts you on. On "good" days, when the number is lower than expected, you feel validated, even euphoric. But that high is fleeting, and it's always followed by the fear that tomorrow's weigh-in won't be as kind. On "bad" days, when the number creeps up, it's a one-way ticket to self-loathing, guilt, and shame. You start questioning your worth, your choices, and your progress—all because of a few fucking digits.

And can we talk about how the scale sabotages your ability to listen to your body? Instead of focusing on how you feel—energized, strong, satisfied—you're fixated on what the scale says. You could be making amazing progress in ways the scale can't measure, like improving your stamina, building muscle, or simply feeling more confident in your skin. But if the number doesn't match your expectations, none of that seems to matter. The scale is a thief, robbing you of your ability to celebrate the things that truly count.

So how do you end this toxic relationship? First, you need to physically remove the scale from your life. Hide it, donate it, or smash it with a hammer if that feels cathartic. The point is, get it out of sight and out of mind. You can't break up with something if it's still lurking in your bathroom, tempting you to step on it every morning.

Next, start focusing on non-scale victories (NSVs). These are the wins that have nothing to do with weight and everything to do with how you feel and what your body can do. Maybe you ran a little farther this week, lifted a little heavier, or slept a little better. Maybe you're feeling more confident in your favorite jeans, or you finally nailed that yoga pose you've been working on. These victories are worth celebrating, and they're a hell of a lot more meaningful than a number on a scale.

It's also important to reframe your mindset around progress. Instead of asking, "What does the scale say?" start asking, "How do I feel?" Are you feeling stronger, happier, more energized? Are you enjoying your meals, moving your body in ways that feel good, and living your life without constant guilt or anxiety? These are the questions that actually matter—not whether you've lost or gained a pound.

Breaking up with the scale also means redefining success on your own terms. Diet culture loves to tell us that success is all about weight loss, but that's a load of crap. Success can be whatever you want it to be— feeling more confident, having more energy, or simply being kinder to yourself. You get to decide what progress looks like, and you don't need a scale to validate it.

Finally, give yourself permission to let go of the guilt. You're not a bad person for stepping on the scale, and you're not a bad person for deciding to break up with it. This is about reclaiming your power and refusing to let a piece of metal dictate your happiness. It's about choosing to live a life that's free from the constant judgment of diet culture and its toxic tools.

Breaking up with your daily weigh-in isn't easy, especially if you've been relying on the scale for validation for years. But it's one of the most liberating things you can do for your mental and physical health. You are so much more than a number, and it's time to start living like it.

The scale doesn't define you. It doesn't measure your worth, your beauty, or your potential. It's just a tool—a shitty, unreliable, manipulative tool that you don't need in your life. So kick it to the curb, celebrate your non-scale victories, and start living a life that's free from its bullshit. Because you deserve better, and the scale deserves to be left in the dust.

Celebrating Non-Scale Wins: Like Not Throwing Your Scale Out the Window This Week

Let's take a moment to celebrate the victories that actually matter—the ones diet culture doesn't give a shit about because they don't fit neatly into a calorie-counting app or a number on the scale. These are the *non-scale wins*, the glorious little triumphs that remind you life is about more than obsessing over your gravitational pull on a piece of metal. And hey, if you didn't chuck your scale out the window this week, that's already a fucking win in my book.

First off, let's talk about what a non-scale win even is. It's any success, no matter how small, that has nothing to do with your weight. Maybe you tried a new recipe and didn't burn the house down. Maybe you said "fuck it" and wore the shorts, cellulite be damned. Maybe you walked up a flight of stairs without feeling like you needed an oxygen tank, or you had pizza for dinner and didn't spend the next three hours spiraling into food guilt. These moments might seem small, but they're big deals—and they deserve to be celebrated like the victories they are.

Diet culture doesn't want you to focus on non-scale wins because they don't feed into its bullshit narrative. It wants you to believe that the only progress worth celebrating is weight loss. But here's the truth: weight is just one tiny piece of the puzzle, and it's not even the most important one. The real wins are the ones that make you feel stronger, happier, and more like your badass self—and those wins don't come with a number attached.

Let's start with the physical wins. These are the moments where your body reminds you what a fucking rockstar it is. Maybe you've been hitting the gym, and suddenly you can lift a little heavier or run a little farther. Maybe you've been practicing yoga, and you finally nailed that downward dog without feeling like you were going to pass out. Or maybe you're just feeling more energized, more flexible, or less like your body hates you when you wake up in the morning. These are the wins that matter—not the number on the scale.

And let's not forget the mental wins. These are the moments where you told diet culture to shove it and did something that made you happy. Maybe you skipped the guilt trip and ate the ice cream. Maybe you looked in the mirror and decided to focus on what you love about your body instead of what you want to change. Maybe you stopped comparing yourself to some airbrushed Instagram influencer and realized you're pretty fucking awesome just the way you are. These mental victories are priceless, and they're worth celebrating every damn day.

Food wins are another big one. Diet culture has spent so long fucking with our relationship with food that even the simplest victories feel monumental. Maybe you tried intuitive eating for the first time and didn't overthink every bite. Maybe you cooked a meal that actually tasted good instead of choking down another sad salad. Or maybe you let yourself enjoy dessert without calculating how many burpees it would take to "burn it off." These are the moments where you're reclaiming your relationship with food, and that's worth raising a goddamn toast to.

Non-scale wins also include the moments where you put yourself out there and lived your life without letting diet culture hold you back.

Maybe you wore the swimsuit, even though you felt nervous as hell. Maybe you danced like a lunatic at a party and didn't give a fuck what anyone thought. Maybe you went out to eat with friends and ordered what you actually wanted instead of what felt "safe." These are the moments where you're choosing joy, freedom, and connection over bullshit rules—and that's fucking powerful.

The beauty of non-scale wins is that they're deeply personal. They're not about meeting someone else's expectations or living up to some arbitrary standard—they're about what matters to *you*. Maybe your win is as simple as drinking enough water for the first time in weeks. Maybe it's choosing to rest when your body needed it, instead of forcing yourself to work out. Maybe it's deleting the calorie-counting app that was sucking the life out of you. Whatever it is, it's your win, and it's worth celebrating.

Now, let's talk about how to actually celebrate these wins. First and foremost, acknowledge them. Diet culture loves to downplay anything that isn't weight loss, so it's up to you to give your wins the credit they deserve. Write them down, say them out loud, or share them with a friend who gets it. The more you celebrate your non-scale victories, the more you'll realize just how much progress you're making—progress that actually matters.

Next, find ways to reward yourself that have nothing to do with food or exercise. Maybe it's treating yourself to a bubble bath, buying that outfit you've been eyeing, or taking yourself on a solo date to your favorite coffee shop. Rewards don't have to be extravagant—they just have to feel good. And no, you don't need to "earn" them by hitting some arbitrary goal. You're allowed to treat yourself just for existing.

It's also important to reframe how you think about progress. Diet culture has trained us to see progress as linear—a straight line from "before" to "after." But real progress is messy, nonlinear, and full of ups and downs. It's the moments where you take two steps forward and one step back, and that's okay. Progress isn't about perfection—it's about persistence.

Finally, surround yourself with people who celebrate your wins with you. Whether it's a supportive friend, a therapist, or an online community, having people in your corner makes all the difference. These are the people who will cheer you on when you're kicking ass and remind you of your worth when you're struggling. And let's be honest: everyone deserves a hype squad.

Celebrating non-scale wins is about more than just patting yourself on the back—it's about reclaiming your relationship with yourself and your body. It's about choosing to focus on what truly matters, instead of what diet culture wants you to obsess over. So go ahead and celebrate every little victory, from wearing the shorts to smashing your scale. Because you're doing the damn thing, and that's worth celebrating.

Non-scale wins are the real MVPs of progress. They're the moments that remind you you're more than a number, and you're so much stronger, braver, and more badass than diet culture ever gave you credit for. So keep smashing those wins, keep celebrating yourself, and keep living your best fucking life. You've earned it.

Chapter 5

When Diet Culture Wears a Disguise

"Wellness" My Ass: How Diet Culture Put On Yoga Pants and Called Itself Self-Care

Let's talk about how diet culture went and pulled a sneaky little makeover. Somewhere along the line, it realized that words like "diet" and "weight loss" were starting to make people roll their eyes harder than a teenager grounded on a Saturday night. So what did it do? It threw on a pair of overpriced yoga pants, lit a eucalyptus candle, and rebranded itself as "wellness." And just like that, a wolf in sheep's clothing strutted onto the scene, peddling the same toxic bullshit but now wrapped in pastel hues and the hashtag #selfcare.

At first glance, "wellness" seems harmless, even positive. Who doesn't want to be well, right? But dig a little deeper, and you'll find that wellness culture is just diet culture in disguise. It's the same restrictive rules, the same obsession with thinness, and the same guilt-ridden marketing—just with a shiny new coat of paint. It's like your shitty ex showing up in a nice suit, claiming they've changed. Spoiler alert: they haven't.

Take a stroll through Instagram, and you'll see what I mean. Influencers posting pictures of their green juices with captions like, "Just cleansing my body and soul!" Brands selling detox teas that promise to "flatten your tummy" and "reduce bloat." Wellness retreats offering yoga classes and vegan meals in the name of "finding balance." It's all the same crap, just dressed up in a prettier package.

The problem with wellness culture is that it weaponizes self-care. It takes something that's supposed to make you feel good—like taking a bath, going for a walk, or enjoying a good meal—and turns it into another way to control your body and your life. Suddenly, self-care isn't about listening to your needs or treating yourself with kindness. It's about eating "clean," exercising religiously, and posting about it so everyone knows how "balanced" and "dedicated" you are.

Let's talk about the term "clean eating," which wellness culture loves to throw around like confetti. At first glance, it sounds innocent—who doesn't want to eat food that's "clean"? But think about what it implies. If some foods are "clean," then others must be "dirty," right? And if you eat those "dirty" foods, what does that make you? It's a subtle but powerful way of making you feel guilty for enjoying a slice of pizza or a donut, as if you've somehow failed as a human being for eating something that didn't come straight from the earth.

And don't even get me started on detoxes. Wellness culture is obsessed with the idea that your body is some kind of toxic wasteland in need of a good scrubbing. "Flush out the toxins!" they scream, while waving bottles of overpriced juice in your face. But here's the truth: your liver and kidneys are already detoxing your body like the hardworking MVPs they are. They don't need help from a $12 bottle of celery juice or a tea that's basically a laxative in disguise.

Then there's the wellness obsession with "natural" everything. Natural foods, natural beauty products, natural deodorant. While there's nothing wrong with wanting fewer chemicals in your life, wellness culture takes it to extremes, making you feel like a failure if you dare to eat a processed granola bar or use shampoo that isn't handmade by a free-spirited artisan named Moonbeam. It's exhausting, expensive, and completely unnecessary.

And let's not forget how wellness culture co-opts fitness. Exercise, in its purest form, is about moving your body in ways that feel good and make you happy. But wellness culture turns it into a performance. It's not enough to work out—you have to work out *right*. You need the perfect outfit, the perfect playlist, and a post-workout smoothie that costs more than your electric bill. And heaven forbid you work out for fun instead of to "sculpt" or "tone" your body.

The most insidious thing about wellness culture is how it convinces you it's all for your own good. It's not about weight loss, they say—it's about health! It's not about being thin—it's about balance! But scratch the surface, and you'll find the same old diet culture messaging underneath. Be smaller. Eat less. Control your body. It's all about selling you the idea that you're not good enough as you are, and that you need their products, programs, and approval to be worthy.

So how do we fight back against wellness culture? First, start questioning everything. The next time someone tries to sell you a detox, a cleanse, or a meal plan, ask yourself: Who's benefiting from this? What are they trying to sell me? And most importantly, do I really need this, or am I being manipulated by marketing?

Second, reclaim self-care on your own terms. True self-care isn't about conforming to wellness culture's bullshit—it's about doing what makes you feel good, without guilt or shame. If that means eating a salad, great. If it means eating a burger, also great. Self-care is about listening to your body and giving it what it needs, not following someone else's rules.

Third, start focusing on how you feel instead of how you look. Wellness culture loves to make it all about appearances—your weight, your skin, your "glow." But real health is about feeling strong, energized, and happy in your own skin. It's about being able to live your life without constantly worrying about whether you're doing enough to meet someone else's definition of "wellness."

Finally, surround yourself with people and messages that celebrate you as you are. Unfollow the influencers who make you feel like shit, and start following accounts that promote body positivity, food freedom, and real self-care. Build a community that supports you in living your best, most authentic life—not one that tries to sell you snake oil.

"Wellness" might be the new face of diet culture, but it doesn't have to run your life. You're smarter than their marketing, stronger than their guilt trips, and more than enough just as you are. So throw on whatever deodorant you want, eat the processed granola bar, and enjoy the freedom of living your life without wellness culture's bullshit. Because self-care isn't about detoxing your body—it's about detoxing your mind from the lies they've been feeding you.

Guilt-Language Bingo: Spotting Words Like "Cheat Meal" and "Detox" for the BS They Are

Let's play a game, shall we? It's called Guilt-Language Bingo, and it's designed to help you spot the manipulative, shame-filled bullshit that diet culture sprinkles into our everyday language. Words like "cheat meal," "detox," "clean eating," and "guilt-free" are everywhere, slipping into our vocab like that annoying neighbor who always shows up uninvited. These phrases might seem harmless at first, but they're loaded with judgment, guilt, and an unspoken message: You're not good enough as you are. Well, fuck that noise. It's time to call out these linguistic landmines for the toxic crap they really are.

Let's start with "cheat meal," one of diet culture's favorite terms. On the surface, it sounds like a harmless way to describe indulging in your favorite foods. But think about what it's actually saying. "Cheat" implies you're breaking the rules, doing something wrong, or being naughty. It turns a perfectly normal act—eating food you enjoy—into a moral failing. Like you've committed some kind of culinary sin that needs to be atoned for with extra burpees or a week of salads. Newsflash: you're not "cheating" when you eat pizza or cake. You're just fucking eating.

And then there's "detox," the buzzword that refuses to die. Every time you turn around, someone's trying to sell you a detox tea, a detox juice cleanse, or a detox diet that promises to "flush out toxins" and "reset your body." But here's the truth: your body is already detoxing itself, every second of every day. That's literally what your liver and kidneys are for. They don't need help from a bottle of overpriced green sludge or a tea that will have you sprinting to the bathroom every 10 minutes. The only thing you're flushing out with a detox is your money.

"Clean eating" is another one that needs to fuck right off. At first glance, it seems like a positive concept—who doesn't want to eat "clean," right? But the problem with this term is that it implies there's such a thing as "dirty" eating. Like if you dare to enjoy a slice of pizza or a bag of chips, you're somehow polluting your body. It's food, not a moral dilemma. You don't need to "cleanse" yourself after eating fries, and you're not a better person because you chose quinoa over rice. Food doesn't have morals, and neither does your plate.

Then we have the insidious phrase "guilt-free." You've seen it plastered on everything from ice cream to granola bars, promising you can enjoy these foods without the crushing weight of shame. But here's the thing: why the fuck should food come with guilt in the first place? Guilt is for things like forgetting your friend's birthday or accidentally stepping on your dog's tail—not eating a cookie. The fact that we need a term like "guilt-free" is a testament to how deeply diet culture has fucked with our relationship with food.

"Indulgent" is another sneaky little bastard. It's a word that diet culture uses to describe foods that are rich, decadent, or—heaven forbid— calorie-dense. It frames these foods as rare treats, something you can only enjoy occasionally and with a side of guilt. But let's be real: life is too short to eat nothing but plain chicken and steamed broccoli. If you want a brownie, eat the damn brownie. You don't need to treat it like a forbidden treasure or ration it like it's the last piece of chocolate on Earth.

And let's not forget the ultimate diet culture classic: "guilt trip." You eat something "off plan," and suddenly that little voice in your head is screaming about how you've ruined everything. "You shouldn't have eaten that," it says. "Now you'll have to work twice as hard tomorrow." It's a full-blown guilt-tripping spiral, designed to make you feel like shit for doing something as basic and necessary as eating. But here's the thing: food guilt is a scam. It's a tool diet culture uses to keep you in line, and it's time to stop falling for it.

So how do you fight back against guilt-language? First, start paying attention to the words you use and hear around food. Every time you catch yourself or someone else using a phrase like "cheat meal" or "guilt-free," call it out for the bullshit it is. Replace these toxic terms with language that's neutral, positive, or downright celebratory. Instead of "cheat meal," say "favorite meal." Instead of "guilt-free," say "fucking delicious." You get the idea.

Second, stop moralizing your food choices. Eating a salad doesn't make you a saint, and eating a burger doesn't make you a sinner. They're just choices, and they're both valid. Food is not a test of your character, and you're not a better or worse person based on what's on your plate.

Third, give yourself permission to enjoy your food without judgment. If you're eating something you love, savor it. Don't waste a single bite on guilt, shame, or regret. Life is too short to spend it apologizing for your cravings.

Finally, start surrounding yourself with messages and people that support a healthy, positive relationship with food. Follow accounts that promote food freedom, body positivity, and self-compassion. Unfollow the ones that make you feel like shit. Build a community that celebrates food as a source of joy, nourishment, and connection—not as a tool for control or punishment.

Guilt-language is diet culture's sneakiest weapon, but you're smarter than their bullshit. By calling out these toxic terms, replacing them with empowering language, and celebrating your relationship with food, you can take back your power and start living your life on your own terms. So go ahead, play Guilt-Language Bingo, spot the bullshit, and tell it to fuck off. Because you deserve better than their lies, and food deserves better than their shame.

Social Media's Diet Cult: How to Unfollow Karen and Her Kale Smoothies

Let's take a stroll through the cesspool of comparison, shall we? I'm talking about social media—the unofficial headquarters of diet culture's propaganda machine. You know the scene: your feed is flooded with influencers who look like they've never eaten a carb in their lives, posting pictures of kale smoothies, "clean" meals, and gym selfies with captions like, "No excuses!" or "#Blessed to be working on my fitness!" It's a never-ending parade of unattainable body standards, guilt-inducing food photos, and enough bullshit to fertilize an entire farm. It's time to unfollow Karen and her kale smoothies and take back your mental health.

Let's start with Karen—the ultimate social media archetype of diet culture. Karen isn't just a person; she's a phenomenon. She's the one who makes you feel like shit for eating a cookie while she's out here blending spinach and spirulina into a glass and calling it breakfast. Karen thrives on "motivational" posts that are really just thinly veiled guilt trips. "If I can do it, so can you!" she chirps, while doing burpees in a matching pastel workout set. The subtext? "If you're not doing it, you're a lazy piece of crap."

Social media Karen is the queen of toxic positivity. She posts before-and-after photos with captions like, "I didn't like who I was, so I changed!" Translation: "I used to be fat and sad, but now I'm thin and happy, and you should be too." Never mind that happiness isn't something you can Photoshop into existence or that weight loss doesn't automatically solve all your problems. Karen doesn't care about nuance—she cares about likes, shares, and being the patron saint of #Fitspo.

Then there's Karen's kale smoothies, which are basically the diet culture mascot. They're green, they're gross, and they're held up as the ultimate symbol of health. But here's the thing: drinking kale isn't going to magically transform your life. It's not going to make you a better person, and it's certainly not going to taste good. Kale smoothies are just another way for Karen to flex her "discipline" while you're over here wondering if it's socially acceptable to eat pizza for breakfast. (Spoiler: it is.)

Social media diet culture doesn't stop with Karen. It's a whole goddamn cult, complete with its own language, rituals, and high priests. The hashtags alone are enough to make you want to throw your phone into the nearest body of water. #CleanEating. #Detox. #CheatDay. #NoPainNoGain. They're plastered on every post like a badge of honor, reinforcing the idea that your worth is tied to how much kale you can choke down or how many burpees you can suffer through.

And let's not ignore the airbrushed, filtered-to-hell images that dominate your feed. These aren't just unrealistic—they're fucking lies. Karen doesn't wake up looking like that. Karen doesn't even look like that. But every time you scroll past her perfectly posed selfies, your brain starts whispering, "Why don't I look like that? What's wrong with me?" The answer? Nothing. Absolutely nothing is wrong with you. What's wrong is a culture that prioritizes appearances over authenticity and profits over mental health.

Social media diet culture also loves to slide into your DMs with unsolicited advice and product pitches. "Hey, girl! I noticed you're trying to be healthier! Have you heard about our detox tea/weight loss shake/waist trainer?" These pyramid-scheme Karens are out here pretending to care about your well-being while really just trying to line their pockets. Newsflash: if someone's health advice comes with a promo code, you probably shouldn't take it.

So how do you break free from the cult of social media diet culture? First, start curating your feed like it's your personal sanctuary. Unfollow Karen and anyone else who makes you feel like shit about yourself. If their posts leave you feeling guilty, inadequate, or like you need to buy something to "fix" yourself, hit that unfollow button like it owes you money.

Next, start following accounts that promote body positivity, food freedom, and self-compassion. Fill your feed with voices that celebrate diversity, challenge diet culture, and remind you that you're fucking awesome just as you are. The more you surround yourself with these messages, the easier it'll be to drown out the noise of diet culture.

It's also time to set some boundaries with social media. Limit how much time you spend scrolling, and remember that most of what you see isn't real. Karen's life isn't as perfect as her feed makes it seem, and her kale smoothies aren't going to make you any happier. Take a step back, reconnect with reality, and remind yourself that your worth isn't measured in likes or followers.

And let's talk about resisting the urge to compare. Comparison is the lifeblood of social media diet culture—it thrives on making you feel like you're not enough. But the truth is, you're not supposed to look like anyone else. You're supposed to look like *you*. Stop comparing your behind-the-scenes to someone else's highlight reel and start celebrating the unique badass that you are.

Finally, start calling out the bullshit when you see it. If someone posts a "motivational" caption that's really just a guilt trip, don't be afraid to say, "Actually, no thanks." If Karen starts hawking detox teas in her stories, send her a link to an article about how detoxes are a scam. The more we challenge diet culture on social media, the less power it has to manipulate and control us.

Social media's diet cult is one of the most insidious parts of modern diet culture, but it doesn't have to run your life. You have the power to curate your feed, protect your mental health, and take back your joy. So unfollow Karen, block her kale smoothies, and start building a social media experience that uplifts you instead of tearing you down. Because you deserve better than their bullshit, and your happiness is worth more than their likes.

Chapter 6

Love Your Body, Even If It's a Pain in the Ass Sometimes

Body Neutrality: A Realistic Option When You're Feeling Blah—Because Loving It Every Day Isn't Required

Let's cut the bullshit for a second: loving your body every single day is hard as fuck. Some days you wake up, look in the mirror, and feel like a goddamn rockstar. Other days, you catch a glimpse of yourself in a poorly lit dressing room and spiral into a pit of self-loathing because your thighs dared to exist. It's a rollercoaster, and anyone who tells you they're 100% in love with their body all the time is either lying or heavily medicated. But here's the thing: you don't have to love your body every day. You just have to stop hating it.

Enter body neutrality—the chill, no-pressure cousin of body positivity. It's the philosophy that says, "Hey, your body is cool because it keeps you alive. You don't have to love it, but maybe just don't be a dick to it, okay?" Body neutrality is all about focusing on what your body *does* rather than what it *looks* like. It's like the middle finger to diet culture's endless obsession with appearances, and honestly, it's a breath of fresh fucking air.

So, what does body neutrality actually look like in practice? It starts with letting go of the pressure to always feel great about your body. Diet culture has warped body positivity into this toxic positivity nightmare where you're supposed to wake up every day singing "I'm Sexy and I Know It" while staring lovingly at your reflection. But let's be real: some days, you just feel blah. Maybe you're bloated, tired, or dealing with a breakout that makes you want to crawl back under the covers. And that's okay. You're allowed to have days where you're not head-over-heels for your body.

Body neutrality is about taking the focus off your body's appearance and putting it on its function. Instead of fixating on whether your thighs look "too big" in those jeans, remind yourself that those thighs let you squat, dance, or run up the stairs when you're late for work. Instead of obsessing over your stomach's lack of definition, think about how it digests food and gives you the energy to get through your day. Your body is a fucking miracle, and it's doing its best to keep you alive— maybe cut it some slack.

Let's talk about the language we use to describe our bodies. Diet culture thrives on harsh, critical language—words like "flabby," "gross," and "problem areas" that make you feel like your body is some kind of fixer-upper project. Body neutrality, on the other hand, is all about using neutral, factual language. Instead of saying, "Ugh, my arms are so flabby," try saying, "My arms help me lift things." Instead of saying, "My stomach is disgusting," try saying, "My stomach digests food." It might feel weird at first, but it's a hell of a lot better than dragging yourself down with negativity.

Body neutrality also means accepting that your body isn't perfect—and that's okay. Perfection is a myth perpetuated by Photoshop, filters, and a billion-dollar beauty industry that thrives on making you feel inadequate. Your body has scars, stretch marks, and weird little quirks that make it uniquely yours. Embracing body neutrality means recognizing that those so-called "flaws" are just part of being human. They're not bad—they just *are*.

One of the biggest hurdles to body neutrality is the constant barrage of diet culture bullshit telling you that your body isn't good enough. Everywhere you look, there are ads, influencers, and social media posts screaming, "Fix this! Tone that! Slim down here!" It's exhausting, and it makes it damn near impossible to just exist in your body without feeling like you need to change it. The first step to fighting back is to stop giving those voices so much power. Unfollow the influencers, block the ads, and start filling your life with people and messages that celebrate you as you are.

Another key part of body neutrality is treating your body with kindness, even when you're not feeling great about it. That means feeding it when it's hungry, resting when it's tired, and moving it in ways that feel good—not as punishment, but as a celebration of what your body can do. It also means wearing clothes that make you feel comfortable and confident, rather than squeezing yourself into something just because it's "flattering."

Let's talk about movement, because diet culture loves to turn exercise into a punishment for eating. Body neutrality flips that script. Instead of working out to burn calories or "earn" your food, move your body because it feels good. Dance, stretch, swim, lift, or just take a leisurely walk—whatever brings you joy and makes your body feel alive. Exercise shouldn't be a chore or a punishment; it should be a way to connect with your body and celebrate its strength.

One of the most liberating things about body neutrality is that it frees up so much mental energy. When you're not constantly worrying about how your body looks, you can focus on all the other amazing things you are and do. You can invest your time and energy into your passions, your relationships, and your dreams instead of wasting it on self-criticism. It's like hitting the mute button on that little voice in your head that's always nitpicking your reflection.

Body neutrality also means recognizing that your worth isn't tied to your appearance. You're not more valuable because you're thin, and you're not less valuable because you're not. Your worth comes from who you are as a person—your kindness, your humor, your intelligence, and the unique spark that only you bring to the world. Your body is just the vehicle that carries you through life, and it deserves respect, not judgment.

Practicing body neutrality takes time, especially if you've spent years steeped in diet culture's toxic messaging. But every small step you take—every moment of kindness, every shift in perspective, every time you choose to focus on what your body does instead of how it looks—is a victory. It's a journey, not a destination, and you don't have to get it right every day.

Body neutrality is about finding peace with your body, even when you don't love it. It's about recognizing that your body is good enough just as it is, and that you don't have to spend your life trying to change it. So take a deep breath, give yourself a break, and start treating your body with the respect it deserves. Because even when it's a pain in the ass, your body is still pretty fucking amazing.

Beauty Standards Are Bullsh*t: Who Decided Hip Dips Were a Thing to Hate?

Let's get this out of the way: beauty standards are complete and utter bullshit. They're arbitrary, ever-changing, and designed to make you feel like shit so you'll spend money chasing some unattainable ideal. And hip dips? That's just the latest thing some bored asshole in a boardroom decided to slap a "problem" label on so they could sell you creams, workouts, and Spanx to "fix" it. Newsflash: you don't need fixing. Beauty standards are the real problem here, not your perfectly normal, perfectly fine body.

Let's talk about hip dips, the current target of diet culture's obsession. For those of you lucky enough to be unfamiliar with this nonsense, hip dips are the little inward curves between your hips and thighs. That's it. They're not a disease, a deformity, or even something new—they're just a part of human anatomy. And yet, thanks to some shitty beauty trend, people are now freaking out over a body part most of us didn't even think twice about until Instagram got involved.

Hip dips are just the tip of the iceberg when it comes to the insanity of beauty standards. One decade, everyone's trying to look like a Victoria's Secret model, starving themselves to achieve that waifish figure. The next, it's all about big asses and tiny waists, with people shelling out thousands for Brazilian butt lifts and waist trainers. And now, apparently, we're supposed to have smooth, seamless curves with no dips, bumps, or wrinkles. Are you fucking kidding me?

Here's the thing about beauty standards: they're designed to be unattainable. If everyone could easily achieve them, the industries that profit off your insecurities wouldn't make a dime. That's why they keep moving the goalposts, inventing new "flaws," and convincing you that you're not good enough as you are. First, it was cellulite. Then it was stretch marks. Now it's hip dips. What's next? Elbow wrinkles? Toe shapes?

The real kicker is that beauty standards aren't even based on reality. They're created by marketers, Photoshopped to hell and back, and promoted by influencers who are either genetically blessed, surgically enhanced, or both. Nobody actually looks like the airbrushed, filtered images you see on social media, not even the people in the photos. And yet, we're all out here comparing ourselves to these fake-ass standards and feeling like failures because we don't measure up.

Let's not ignore the role of social media in perpetuating this bullshit. Platforms like Instagram and TikTok are breeding grounds for toxic beauty trends, with influencers constantly pushing the latest "must-have" look. They'll post videos of themselves contouring their hip dips, using shapewear to smooth out their curves, or doing "targeted exercises" to get rid of a body part that isn't even a problem. And the worst part? They frame it as "self-care" or "body positivity," as if masking your natural shape is somehow empowering. Spoiler alert: it's not.

The beauty industry, of course, is loving every second of this. They're out here making billions off your insecurities, selling you creams, serums, and workout plans to "fix" the things they told you were wrong with you. They don't actually give a shit about your health or happiness—they just want your money. And the more insecure you feel, the more money they make. It's a vicious cycle, and it's time to break the fuck out of it.

So how do we fight back against beauty standards? First, stop giving a shit about what society says you're supposed to look like. You weren't put on this earth to be a walking mannequin for someone else's idea of beauty. Your worth isn't determined by your body shape, your skin texture, or whether or not you have hip dips. You're a whole-ass human being with talents, passions, and a personality that can't be measured in inches or pounds.

Next, start calling out the bullshit when you see it. If a brand tries to sell you a product to "fix" a body part you didn't even know was a problem, call them out. If an influencer posts a video promoting some toxic beauty trend, unfollow their ass. The more we push back against this nonsense, the less power it has to control us.

It's also time to start celebrating real bodies. Bodies with hip dips, cellulite, stretch marks, scars, and all the other things beauty standards tell us to hate. Your body tells your story, and every so-called "flaw" is a chapter in that story. They're not imperfections—they're badges of honor that prove you've lived, laughed, and experienced life.

Another way to fight back is to curate your media consumption. Follow accounts and brands that promote body positivity, diversity, and authenticity. Fill your feed with images of people who look like you, instead of the unattainable ideals that diet culture pushes. The more you surround yourself with these messages, the easier it'll be to drown out the noise of beauty standards.

Finally, start practicing radical self-acceptance. This doesn't mean you have to love every part of your body every day—that's not realistic. But it does mean respecting your body for what it is and refusing to let society's bullshit make you feel bad about it. It means looking in the mirror and saying, "Yeah, I have hip dips. So fucking what?"

Beauty standards are bullsh*t, plain and simple. They're designed to make you feel like you're not enough so that someone else can profit off your insecurities. But you don't have to play their game. You're already enough, just as you are. So embrace your hip dips, your cellulite, your stretch marks, and every other thing society tries to make you hate. Because at the end of the day, the only opinion that matters is your own—and you're fucking perfect just the way you are.

Treat Yo' Self Right: Self-Care Without a Calorie Count or Instagram Filter

Let's talk about self-care—the kind that doesn't come with a price tag, a calorie count, or an Instagram filter. Not the faux "self-care" that diet culture has hijacked and rebranded to sell you overpriced detox teas, face masks, and gym memberships. I'm talking about real, honest-to-fuck self-care. The kind that makes you feel good without a side of guilt or a spreadsheet to track your macros. Because newsflash: self-care is supposed to be about taking care of *yourself*, not turning your life into a Pinterest board.

Diet culture's version of self-care is like the shitty ex who always "forgets" their wallet at dinner—it promises a lot but delivers nothing. It convinces you that self-care is all about being productive, achieving goals, and sticking to a routine. Drink your green juice, wake up at 5 a.m. to meditate, and log your 12,000 steps before breakfast, because apparently, relaxation is just another thing to hustle for. But here's the truth: real self-care isn't about earning your rest or justifying your indulgences. It's about giving yourself what you need, no strings attached.

First of all, self-care does *not* have to be Instagram-worthy. You don't need to light a candle, set up a bubble bath, and stage an elaborate photo shoot just to prove you're taking care of yourself. Sometimes, self-care looks like sitting on the couch in your oldest, rattiest sweatpants, eating pizza straight out of the box while binge-watching your favorite show. And guess what? That's fucking valid.

Real self-care is messy, imperfect, and deeply personal. It's about listening to what your body and mind need, not what society says you should want. Maybe you need to skip the gym and sleep in. Maybe you need to cancel plans and have a solo night in. Maybe you need to scream-sing to angry breakup songs in your car, even though you're not even in a breakup. Whatever it is, self-care is about doing what feels good for *you*—not what looks good to other people.

One of the biggest lies diet culture tells us is that self-care has to be productive. That every act of rest or relaxation has to somehow contribute to your goals, whether it's burning calories, detoxing your body, or clearing your mind. But real self-care doesn't have to achieve anything. It doesn't have to make you thinner, fitter, or more Zen. Sometimes, it's just about existing—about taking a goddamn break without feeling guilty for it.

And let's talk about guilt, because diet culture loves to sprinkle that shit onto everything. Take a day off from working out? Guilt. Eat a dessert because you fucking wanted it? Double guilt. Spend an afternoon doing absolutely nothing? Guilt with a side of shame. But here's the thing: you don't owe anyone productivity, least of all yourself. Rest is not lazy.

Indulgence is not sinful. Taking care of yourself is not something you need to apologize for.

Self-care also doesn't have to be expensive. You don't need to drop hundreds of dollars on spa treatments, yoga retreats, or organic candles that smell like freshly cut grass. Sure, those things can be nice, but they're not the be-all and end-all of self-care. Sometimes, self-care is as simple as taking a nap, calling a friend, or saying "no" to something you don't want to do. It's not about spending money—it's about spending time and energy on yourself.

Another lie diet culture loves to tell is that self-care always has to be healthy. That every act of relaxation or indulgence should somehow contribute to your physical well-being. But guess what? Sometimes, the healthiest thing you can do is eat a cheeseburger, skip the gym, and spend the entire day in bed. Self-care isn't about following rules—it's about breaking them when they're no longer serving you.

Let's also debunk the myth that self-care is selfish. Taking care of yourself isn't selfish—it's necessary. You can't pour from an empty cup, and you're not going to be much help to anyone else if you're running on fumes. By prioritizing your own needs, you're not just taking care of yourself—you're making yourself better equipped to show up for the people you care about.

So what does real self-care look like? It's different for everyone, but here are a few ideas to get you started.

First, give yourself permission to rest. Whether it's taking a nap, sleeping in, or just lying on the couch doing absolutely nothing, rest is one of the most underrated forms of self-care. Your body and mind need downtime to recharge, and there's nothing lazy or indulgent about giving it to them.

Second, indulge in the things that make you happy, even if they're not "healthy" or "productive." Eat the cake. Drink the wine. Buy the shoes. Life is too short to deny yourself the things that bring you joy.

Third, set boundaries and stick to them. Saying "no" is one of the most powerful forms of self-care, especially when it means protecting your time, energy, and mental health. You don't have to explain yourself or justify your choices—just say "no" and move on.

Fourth, find ways to move your body that feel good, not punishing. Dance, stretch, swim, walk, or do absolutely nothing—it's all valid. The key is to focus on what makes you feel alive and connected to your body, not what burns the most calories or sculpts your abs.

Fifth, connect with the people who lift you up. Self-care isn't always a solo act—sometimes, it's about spending time with friends, family, or your chosen community. Surround yourself with people who support and celebrate you, and don't waste your energy on those who don't.

Finally, remember that self-care is a practice, not a one-time fix. It's about showing up for yourself every day, in whatever way you can. Some days, that might mean doing something big and luxurious. Other days, it might mean just getting out of bed and brushing your teeth. Both are valid, and both are enough.

Self-care without a calorie count or Instagram filter is the ultimate rebellion against diet culture's toxic bullshit. It's about taking care of yourself on your own terms, without guilt, shame, or a need for validation. So treat yo' self—messily, imperfectly, and unapologetically. Because you fucking deserve it.

Chapter 7

Eat Like a Grown-Ass Human Being

Why Food Rules Are Trash: If You Want a Donut for Breakfast, Fuck It—Have Two

Let's cut to the chase: food rules are bullshit. All of them. Every single one. From "don't eat carbs after 7 p.m." to "you can only have dessert on special occasions," food rules are nothing but arbitrary restrictions designed to make you miserable. They're like that one overbearing aunt at Thanksgiving who judges you for taking a second helping of mashed potatoes—completely unnecessary and full of shit. If you want a donut for breakfast, fuck it—have two. Hell, have three. You're a grown-ass adult, and you don't need anyone's permission to eat what you want.

Food rules are the bread and butter (pun intended) of diet culture. They're how it sneaks into your brain and takes over, turning every meal into a minefield of guilt and anxiety. These rules are dressed up as "guidelines" or "best practices," but let's call them what they really are: tools of control. They're not here to help you—they're here to sell you something, whether it's a diet plan, a cookbook, or a sense of superiority over everyone who dared to eat a slice of cake.

Let's break down some of the most common food rules and why they're absolute trash.

1. "Don't eat carbs."

This one's a classic, right up there with "the dog ate my homework" on the list of all-time bullshit excuses. Carbs are not the enemy. They're not out here plotting your demise or sneaking into your pants to make them tighter. Carbs are just fucking carbs—delicious, satisfying, and absolutely essential for giving your body the energy it needs to function. Telling people not to eat carbs is like telling them not to breathe too much oxygen. It's not just unnecessary; it's fucking ridiculous.

2. "No eating after 7 p.m."

What's supposed to happen after 7 p.m.? Do carbs turn into gremlins? Does your metabolism clock out and leave you high and dry? No, none of that happens. Your body doesn't give a shit what time it is—it just knows when it's hungry. If you're craving a midnight snack, go for it. Your stomach isn't wearing a watch, and you shouldn't be either.

3. "Only eat 'clean' foods."

What does "clean" even mean? Did the kale take a shower before landing on your plate? Did the chicken pass a background check? The term "clean eating" is as vague as it is pretentious. It's just another way for diet culture to make you feel bad about eating a burger or a slice of pizza. Newsflash: your body doesn't have a moral compass. It doesn't care if your food is "clean" or "dirty"—it just wants fuel.

4. "Dessert is only for special occasions."

Who the fuck decided this? If you want dessert, have dessert. You don't need to wait for someone's birthday or an official holiday to enjoy a cookie or a slice of cake. Every day you survive the dumpster fire that is modern life is a special occasion, and you deserve to celebrate accordingly.

5. "Always leave something on your plate."
Why? So you can prove you're not a glutton? So you can signal to the world that you have "self-control"? Leaving food on your plate doesn't make you virtuous—it just makes you hungry. If you're full, stop eating. If you're not, keep going. It's not rocket science.

Food rules are bullshit because they take something that should be simple and joyful—eating—and turn it into a fucking chore. They make you second-guess your instincts, ignore your cravings, and feel guilty for enjoying your food. They're the ultimate joy-killers, and it's time to kick them to the curb.

So how do you break free from food rules? First, start listening to your body instead of the bullshit. Your body is smart—it knows what it needs. If you're hungry, eat. If you're full, stop. If you're craving something sweet, have it. Trust your instincts, because they're a hell of a lot more reliable than some arbitrary set of rules.

Second, stop labeling foods as "good" or "bad." Food is just food. A salad isn't "good," and a donut isn't "bad." They're just different, and they both have a place in your diet. By removing the moral judgment from your food choices, you can start eating with freedom and enjoyment instead of guilt and shame.

Third, start challenging the rules directly. The next time you hear someone say, "You shouldn't eat that," respond with, "Says who?" If you catch yourself thinking, "I shouldn't have this," ask yourself why.

Who decided that eating a donut for breakfast was a crime against humanity? The more you question the rules, the more you'll realize they're completely arbitrary and not worth following.

Fourth, start celebrating your food choices instead of apologizing for them. If you want a donut, savor every fucking bite. If you're craving pasta, make the most indulgent, cheesy, carby masterpiece you can dream up. Stop eating like you're trying to impress someone and start eating like a grown-ass adult who knows what they like.

Finally, give yourself permission to eat for pleasure. Food isn't just fuel—it's culture, connection, and joy. It's Sunday brunch with your friends, birthday cake with your family, and midnight pizza after a night out. These moments matter, and they're worth more than any diet plan or calorie count.

Eating like a grown-ass human being means rejecting the rules, embracing your cravings, and enjoying your food without guilt or shame. It means taking back control from diet culture and deciding for yourself what, when, and how you want to eat. Because at the end of the day, you're the boss of your plate—not the other way around. So eat the donut, skip the bullshit, and live your best fucking life.

Intuitive Eating for Real Life: Listening to Your Body Instead of That Loudmouth in Your Head

Let's be real: the idea of listening to your body when it comes to food sounds like some kind of hippie-dippie bullshit at first. "Oh, just *trust* your body," they say, as if your body isn't the same asshole that once convinced you to eat an entire pint of Ben & Jerry's in one sitting. But here's the thing: intuitive eating isn't about perfection or

enlightenment. It's about shutting up that loudmouth in your head—
the one that's been brainwashed by diet culture—and tuning into what
your body actually needs and wants. Because, surprise! Your body
knows its shit.

First, let's identify that loudmouth in your head. You know the one. It's
the voice that whispers, "You shouldn't eat that," every time you reach
for a cookie. It's the jerk that screams, "You've ruined everything!"
when you dare to eat a meal that isn't kale and quinoa. That voice isn't
you. It's diet culture, sneaking into your brain like an uninvited
houseguest and making itself way too comfortable. And it's time to kick
it the fuck out.

Intuitive eating starts with giving your body the trust it deserves. Your
body is like the friend who always knows the best restaurants—it's got
great taste and solid instincts. The problem is, diet culture has spent
years convincing you to ignore it. "Don't eat when you're hungry," it
says. "Eat what the plan tells you to eat, not what you actually want."
Fuck that. Your body knows when it's hungry, and it knows what it's
hungry for. The key is learning how to listen.

So how do you actually start intuitive eating? It begins with something
revolutionary: eating when you're hungry. Sounds simple, right? But
thanks to diet culture, we've been trained to ignore our hunger cues
and stick to arbitrary schedules instead. Breakfast at 7, lunch at 12,
dinner at 6, snacks only if you're dying. But guess what? Hunger doesn't
give a fuck about your schedule. If you're hungry at 10:30 a.m., eat
something. If you're starving at 3 p.m., have a snack. Your body is not a
clock, and you don't need to wait for permission to feed it.

Next, stop categorizing foods into "good" and "bad." This is one of diet culture's oldest tricks, designed to make you feel like shit every time you eat something that's not a salad. But food doesn't have morals. A donut isn't "bad," and a smoothie isn't "good." They're just different, and they both have a place in your diet. Intuitive eating is about giving yourself unconditional permission to eat all foods, without guilt or judgment.

Let's talk about cravings, because diet culture loves to demonize them. "If you're craving chocolate, it means you're deficient in magnesium," they say. "If you're craving chips, you're probably dehydrated." Bullshit. If you're craving chocolate, it means you want chocolate. If you're craving chips, it means you want chips. Cravings are not the enemy— they're your body's way of telling you what it needs or wants. Ignoring them only makes them louder, so stop fighting and start listening.

Another key part of intuitive eating is learning to stop when you're full. This can be tricky, especially if you've spent years cleaning your plate out of guilt or habit. But intuitive eating is not about finishing everything in front of you—it's about eating until you're satisfied and then stopping. If you're halfway through a burger and you're full, save the rest for later. If you're still hungry after your salad, grab a snack. It's not about rules; it's about balance.

One of the biggest hurdles to intuitive eating is the fear of losing control. Diet culture has convinced us that if we stop following the rules, we'll spiral into chaos and end up eating nothing but pizza and ice cream for the rest of our lives. But here's the truth: your body doesn't want to eat pizza and ice cream forever. Sure, you might go a little wild at first—because let's face it, restriction makes you crazy—but eventually, your cravings will even out. You'll start craving balance, because your body *wants* balance.

Let's not forget about the emotional side of eating. Diet culture loves to shame us for eating our feelings, but sometimes a pint of ice cream really is the answer. Emotional eating isn't inherently bad—it's just one of many ways we cope with stress, sadness, or boredom. The key is to recognize it for what it is and make peace with it, instead of letting it spiral into guilt and shame.

Another crucial aspect of intuitive eating is mindfulness. This doesn't mean you have to light a candle and meditate over your meal, but it does mean paying attention to what you're eating and how it makes you feel. Are you enjoying your food? Does it taste good? Does it satisfy you? These questions can help you reconnect with your body and your hunger cues, making eating a more joyful and intuitive experience.

Finally, remember that intuitive eating is not about perfection. There will be days when you overeat, days when you under-eat, and days when you eat nothing but cereal and wine. And that's okay. Intuitive eating is not a diet—it's a lifelong practice of listening to your body and giving it what it needs. It's about progress, not perfection, and every step you take is a step in the right direction.

Intuitive eating is about breaking free from diet culture's bullshit and learning to trust yourself again. It's about eating like a grown-ass human being—messily, imperfectly, and joyfully. So shut up that loudmouth in your head, tune into your body, and start eating the way nature fucking intended. Because you deserve better than their rules, and your body deserves better than their lies.

Bye-Bye, Food Fear: Why Eating Chocolate Cake Won't Summon the Diet Police

Let's get one thing straight: eating chocolate cake, or pizza, or a damn cheeseburger, is not a crime. There is no secret diet police force hiding in the bushes, ready to arrest you the moment a carb crosses your lips. And yet, thanks to diet culture's relentless fear-mongering, so many of us live in terror of certain foods, as if a single bite might ruin our lives. Well, fuck that. It's time to tell food fear to fuck right off and start eating like the badass human beings we are.

Food fear is one of diet culture's nastiest tricks. It starts small, with innocent-seeming advice like, "Maybe skip dessert tonight" or "Be careful with bread—it's full of empty calories!" But before you know it, you're side-eyeing entire food groups, labeling them as "bad," and feeling like a failure every time you eat them. It's a slippery slope, and at the bottom is a life where every meal feels like a battle. Spoiler alert: that's no way to live.

Let's talk about where this fear comes from. Diet culture loves to frame certain foods as the enemy, warning us that they'll make us fat, unhealthy, or unworthy. Carbs? They'll make you balloon up overnight. Sugar? Practically poison. Fat? Don't even think about it. It's like a bad horror movie where the killer is a plate of spaghetti and meatballs. But here's the truth: no single food is inherently bad for you. It's the *fear* that's toxic, not the food.

Take chocolate cake, for example. Diet culture would have you believe that eating it is some kind of moral failing. "You're being naughty," it whispers. "You'll regret this later." But let's break it down: chocolate cake is just a combination of ingredients—flour, sugar, eggs, cocoa—

that your body knows how to process. It's not an evil, sentient dessert plotting your downfall. It's just a fucking cake, and you're allowed to enjoy it.

The same goes for all the other foods diet culture loves to demonize. Bread is not the devil. Ice cream is not a crime. French fries are not a personal attack. These foods are not out to get you—they're just food. They're meant to be eaten, enjoyed, and savored, not feared. And yet, diet culture has convinced us to view them as ticking time bombs, ready to destroy our health and happiness the moment we indulge.

Food fear doesn't just ruin your relationship with certain foods—it ruins your relationship with *all* food. It turns every meal into a mental chess game, where you're constantly strategizing about what you can and can't eat, how much is "too much," and whether or not you've "earned" your calories for the day. It's exhausting, and it takes all the joy out of eating.

So how do we break free from food fear? First, start challenging the bullshit narratives you've been fed. When diet culture tells you a certain food is "bad," ask yourself why. Who decided this? What's the actual evidence? And most importantly, what happens if you eat it? Nine times out of ten, the answer is "nothing." Eating a donut doesn't make you a bad person. Eating a burger doesn't ruin your progress. And eating chocolate cake definitely doesn't summon the diet police.

Next, start reintroducing the foods you've been avoiding. If you've been afraid of carbs, start with a piece of bread. If sugar's your nemesis, have a scoop of ice cream. Take it slow, and pay attention to how you feel—not in a guilt-ridden, "I'm going to regret this" way, but in a curious, open-minded way. Chances are, you'll realize these foods aren't nearly as scary as diet culture made them out to be.

It's also important to stop labeling foods as "good" or "bad." This black-and-white thinking is the foundation of food fear, and it's completely unnecessary. Food is food. Some foods are more nutrient-dense than others, but that doesn't make them better or worse—it just makes them different. A salad isn't "better" than a pizza—it's just a different choice.

Another key step is to focus on balance instead of restriction. Diet culture loves to tell us we have to choose between being "healthy" and enjoying our favorite foods, but that's a false dichotomy. You can have both. You can eat vegetables and dessert. You can enjoy a green smoothie for breakfast and a burger for dinner. Balance isn't about perfection—it's about variety and moderation.

Let's also address the guilt that often comes with eating so-called "bad" foods. Guilt is diet culture's weapon of choice, designed to keep you in line and make you feel like shit every time you step out of bounds. But here's the thing: guilt has no place at the table. Eating a piece of cake doesn't make you weak, lazy, or undisciplined. It makes you human. So the next time you feel guilt creeping in, tell it to fuck off and take another bite.

Food fear thrives on isolation, so start surrounding yourself with people and messages that celebrate food freedom. Follow accounts that promote intuitive eating, body positivity, and anti-diet culture. Talk to friends who share your values, and share meals with people who enjoy food without judgment. The more you normalize eating all foods without fear, the easier it'll be to break free from diet culture's grip.

Finally, remember that food is supposed to be fun. It's supposed to be a source of pleasure, connection, and creativity, not a cause of stress or shame. Chocolate cake isn't just food—it's a celebration. It's a birthday party, a date night, or a random Tuesday that needed a little sweetness. And you deserve to enjoy it without a side of fear.

Breaking free from food fear isn't easy, especially if you've spent years living under diet culture's rules. But every time you choose to eat without guilt, challenge the bullshit narratives, and trust your body, you're taking a step toward food freedom. And that's something worth celebrating—with chocolate cake, of course.

So go ahead, eat the cake. Order the fries. Enjoy the pizza. Life is too short to let diet culture dictate what you can and can't eat. The diet police don't exist, and even if they did, they can kiss your ass. You're in charge of your plate, your choices, and your happiness. And that's the sweetest victory of all.

Chapter 8

Food Freedom: Your Way, Your Rules

Burn the Rule Book: Forget "Good" or "Bad" Foods and Eat What the Fuck You Want

Let's start with a bonfire, shall we? Grab every diet plan, food journal, and calorie-counting app you've ever used and throw that shit into the flames. Watch it burn, baby, because you're about to liberate yourself from the suffocating bullshit of food rules. Forget "good" or "bad" foods, cheat days, and portion sizes measured with a fucking tablespoon. This is food freedom, and the only rules are your rules.

Diet culture has been playing dictator for way too long, telling us what we can eat, when we can eat it, and how guilty we should feel afterward. It's like having a shitty boss micromanaging your lunch break, except the boss lives in your head and never shuts the fuck up. But here's the thing: food is not the enemy, and you're not a bad person for eating a goddamn cheeseburger. It's time to take back control and start eating like the badass, rule-breaking rebel you are.

The first step to food freedom is ditching the labels. Diet culture loves to slap foods with the "good" or "bad" stamp, turning every meal into a moral dilemma. Salad? Good. French fries? Bad. Kale? Virtuous. Ice cream? Sinful. It's like living in a culinary version of The Scarlet Letter, where every bite you take is judged and ranked. But guess what? Food doesn't have morals, and neither does your plate. A cookie isn't "bad," and a smoothie isn't "good"—they're just fucking food.

Burning the rule book means letting go of the idea that you need permission to eat certain foods. You don't need to "earn" your calories with a workout, and you don't need to "deserve" a treat because you were "good" all week. Your body needs food to survive, and you have every right to eat whatever the hell you want, whenever you want. Period.

Let's talk about cravings, because diet culture loves to make them out to be some kind of personal failing. "If you're craving chocolate, it's because you're weak," they say. "If you're craving chips, it's because you lack discipline." Bullshit. Cravings are your body's way of telling you something, whether it's "I need energy" or "I want something salty and crunchy because life is hard right now." Ignoring your cravings doesn't make them go away—it just makes you miserable. So instead of fighting them, lean the fuck in.

Food freedom is about trusting your body to know what it needs. This might feel weird at first, especially if you've spent years letting diet culture call the shots. But your body is smarter than you think, and it's pretty damn good at telling you what it wants. If you're hungry, eat. If you're full, stop. If you're craving pizza, have pizza. And if you're craving a salad (yes, that's a thing that happens), go for it. The key is listening to your body and giving it what it needs, without judgment or guilt.

One of the most liberating things about food freedom is that it allows you to enjoy your favorite foods without turning them into forbidden fruit. Diet culture loves to create this weird, toxic dynamic where "bad" foods are treated like a guilty pleasure, something you can only have in small doses or on special occasions. But when you give yourself permission to eat whatever the fuck you want, whenever you want, those foods lose their power. They're no longer this magical, unattainable thing—they're just food.

Food freedom also means eating for pleasure, not just survival. Diet culture has reduced eating to a functional, joyless act, like refueling a car. But food is so much more than that. It's connection, culture, celebration, and comfort. It's a hot bowl of soup on a cold day, a birthday cake shared with friends, or a midnight snack that makes you smile. Eating is supposed to be fun, so stop treating it like a chore and start enjoying the hell out of it.

Another key part of food freedom is embracing balance. This doesn't mean sticking to some rigid 80/20 rule or obsessing over "moderation." It means letting go of the all-or-nothing mindset and finding a rhythm that works for you. Maybe one day you eat a green smoothie for breakfast and a pizza for dinner. Maybe another day you snack on chips and then crave a big-ass salad. Balance isn't about perfection—it's about variety, flexibility, and doing what feels good.

Let's not forget about the importance of boundaries, especially when it comes to other people's opinions. Diet culture loves to recruit random assholes as its spokespeople—coworkers, family members, even strangers—who feel entitled to comment on your food choices. "Are you really going to eat that?" they'll ask, with a judgmental side-eye. The answer is yes, you are, and they can kindly fuck off. Your plate is none of their business, and you don't owe anyone an explanation for what you eat.

Food freedom is also about redefining health on your own terms. Diet culture loves to pretend it cares about your health, but let's be real: it's only interested in your weight. True health is so much more than a number on a scale—it's physical, mental, and emotional well-being. It's about feeling strong, energized, and happy, not about fitting into someone else's idea of what you should look like.

Finally, food freedom means giving yourself grace. There will be days when you overeat, days when you under-eat, and days when you eat nothing but cereal and wine. And that's okay. Food freedom is not about being perfect—it's about being human. It's about making peace with your body, your cravings, and your choices, and letting go of the guilt and shame that diet culture tries to shove down your throat.

Burning the rule book and embracing food freedom is one of the most empowering things you can do for yourself. It's about taking back control from diet culture, rejecting its bullshit narratives, and living your life on your own terms. So eat the pizza, order the fries, and enjoy the cake. You're the boss of your plate, and you don't need anyone's permission to eat what the fuck you want.

Eating Out Without Freaking Out: No, You Don't Need to Check the Calories on the Menu

Let's talk about eating out—a glorious experience that diet culture has managed to ruin for way too many of us. Instead of focusing on the joy of trying new dishes, spending time with friends, or indulging in something you didn't have to cook yourself, diet culture turns every restaurant visit into a minefield of guilt, anxiety, and mental math. "How many calories are in that?" "Can I swap the fries for a side of steamed broccoli?" "Is the dressing on the side?" Fuck that noise. Eating out is supposed to be fun, not a goddamn calculus exam.

Here's the thing: you don't need to check the calories on the menu. You don't need to mentally calculate how many minutes of cardio it'll take to "burn off" your meal. And you sure as hell don't need to justify your choices to anyone, including yourself. You're a grown-ass adult, and you're allowed to enjoy your meal without turning it into a guilt-ridden therapy session.

Let's start with the menu itself. Diet culture loves to ruin a good thing by slapping calorie counts all over the place, as if the joy of ordering a burger somehow depends on knowing it's 1,200 calories. But here's the truth: calorie counts are a buzzkill. They take something simple and satisfying—choosing what you want to eat—and turn it into a numbers game. And for what? To make you second-guess your choices and feel like shit before the food even hits the table? No thanks.

If you're at a restaurant with calorie counts on the menu, do yourself a favor and ignore them. Pretend they don't exist. Cover them with your hand if you have to. Order what sounds good, not what has the lowest number next to it. Because guess what? Your body doesn't give a fuck about calorie counts. It cares about feeling nourished, satisfied, and happy.

Diet culture also loves to push the idea that eating out is a "special occasion" that requires some kind of strategy or damage control. You know the drill: "Eat a light lunch to save calories for dinner." "Skip the bread basket so you don't ruin your appetite." "Stick to grilled chicken and salad to stay on track." Fuck all of that. Eating out is not a special occasion—it's a normal part of life. And you don't need a strategy to enjoy it.

Let's talk about the bread basket, because it's been unfairly demonized for far too long. Bread is not the enemy. Bread is a gift. Bread is a warm, fluffy slice of happiness that deserves to be enjoyed without guilt or hesitation. So when the server sets that basket down on the table, don't sit there pretending you're too virtuous to indulge. Grab a piece, slather it in butter, and savor the hell out of it.

One of the biggest hurdles to eating out without freaking out is the fear of judgment. Maybe you're worried about what your friends or family will think if you order the loaded nachos instead of the kale salad. Maybe you're afraid of what the server might think when you ask for extra cheese on your burger. But here's the truth: nobody is judging you as harshly as you're judging yourself. And even if they are, fuck 'em. Your food choices are nobody's business but your own.

And let's not forget about the dreaded "healthy options" section of the menu—a diet culture invention designed to make you feel like shit for wanting something more indulgent. "Oh, you don't want the grilled salmon and steamed veggies? How about the 400-calorie quinoa bowl?" No, Karen, I want the goddamn chicken Alfredo, and I'm going to enjoy every creamy, cheesy bite.

Eating out without freaking out also means letting go of the idea that you need to "earn" or "burn off" your meal. You don't need to justify your order with a pre-dinner workout, and you don't need to punish yourself with an extra-long gym session the next day. Food is not a transaction—it's nourishment, pleasure, and connection. You're allowed to eat for no other reason than because you're hungry and it tastes good.

Let's address the guilt that diet culture loves to serve up as a side dish. Maybe you've ordered something "off-plan." Maybe you've eaten more than you intended. Maybe you're feeling full in a way that diet culture has taught you to associate with failure. But here's the thing: guilt is a useless emotion when it comes to food. It doesn't make you healthier, happier, or more disciplined—it just makes you miserable. So instead of beating yourself up, practice some fucking compassion. You're human. You ate. Move on.

One of the best ways to combat food guilt is to focus on the experience, not the calories. Savor the flavors, enjoy the company, and appreciate the fact that you didn't have to cook or clean up. Eating out is about so much more than the food itself—it's about the memories you're making and the joy you're sharing. Don't let diet culture rob you of that.

If you're still struggling to let go of the diet culture bullshit, try flipping the script. Instead of worrying about what you "should" or "shouldn't" eat, ask yourself what you *want* to eat. What sounds good? What will make you feel satisfied and happy? Trust your instincts—they're a hell of a lot more reliable than diet culture's rules.

And if you need a little extra encouragement, remind yourself that one meal is not going to make or break your health. Your body is resilient, adaptable, and capable of handling a variety of foods. One burger won't ruin your progress, just like one salad won't fix everything. It's the big picture that matters, not a single snapshot.

Eating out without freaking out is about reclaiming the joy, freedom, and connection that food is supposed to bring. It's about shutting out the noise of diet culture, trusting your body, and giving yourself permission to eat what you want without guilt or fear. So order the fries, enjoy the dessert, and toast to living your life on your own terms. Because you fucking deserve it.

Your Food Philosophy: Create Your Own Damn Rules—And Then Break Them

Let's get one thing straight: the only person who gets to decide how you eat is you. Not diet culture, not your mom, not your annoying coworker who won't shut the fuck up about their new juice cleanse. You. Food isn't a one-size-fits-all situation, and it's time to stop living by someone else's bullshit rules. It's time to create your own food philosophy—a set of guidelines that actually work for your life, your body, and your happiness. And the best part? You get to break them whenever the fuck you want.

Creating your own food philosophy starts with flipping a giant middle finger to every diet you've ever been on. Diet culture has spent years trying to shove its rules down your throat: no carbs, no sugar, no fun. It's time to spit that shit out and start fresh. Imagine you're building your own food playbook, one that prioritizes your needs, your cravings, and your joy instead of arbitrary restrictions and guilt. What would that look like?

Step one: throw out the idea of "good" and "bad" foods. This black-and-white thinking is diet culture's bread and butter (pun intended), and it's a recipe for disaster. Labeling foods as "good" or "bad" turns every meal into a moral dilemma, where eating a salad makes you a saint and eating a brownie makes you a sinner. Fuck that noise. Food is just food. Some of it's more nutrient-dense, some of it's more indulgent, and all of it can have a place in your life.

Step two: listen to your body. Your body is smarter than diet culture gives it credit for. It knows when it's hungry, when it's full, and what it's craving. The problem is, diet culture has trained us to ignore those signals and follow its rules instead. It's time to unlearn that shit and start tuning into what your body is telling you. Are you hungry? Eat. Are you full? Stop. Are you craving something salty, sweet, or carby? Go for it. Trust me, your body knows its shit.

Step three: make peace with your cravings. Cravings are not the enemy—they're a normal, healthy part of being human. And no, they're not some kind of moral test designed to measure your willpower. Craving chocolate doesn't mean you're weak, and craving fries doesn't mean you're a failure. It just means you're fucking human. So instead of fighting your cravings, lean into them. Eat what you're craving, enjoy the hell out of it, and then move on with your life.

Step four: focus on balance, not perfection. Diet culture loves to preach about "clean eating" and "staying on track," but life isn't a train, and you're not going to derail it by eating a slice of pizza. Balance isn't about being perfect—it's about making choices that work for you in the moment. Maybe that means eating a green smoothie for breakfast and a burger for dinner. Maybe it means having cake for lunch because it's someone's birthday at work. Whatever it looks like, balance is about flexibility, not rigidity.

Step five: break your own damn rules. Once you've created your food philosophy, don't be afraid to throw it out the window whenever the mood strikes. Your rules are not laws—they're guidelines. If you've decided to prioritize eating vegetables but you're really in the mood for nachos, have the fucking nachos. If your philosophy is all about listening to your body but you just want to eat ice cream for dinner because life is hard and you deserve it, go for it. Your food philosophy should serve you, not the other way around.

Step six: stop giving a shit about what other people think. This is your food philosophy, not theirs. If someone has a problem with the way you eat, that's their problem, not yours. You don't owe anyone an explanation, and you definitely don't owe them an apology. Eat what you want, when you want, and let the haters choke on their judgment.

Step seven: find joy in your food. Diet culture has turned eating into a chore, a punishment, and a source of stress. It's time to take that shit back. Food is supposed to be fun. It's supposed to bring you joy, comfort, and connection. Whether you're savoring a home-cooked meal, indulging in your favorite dessert, or trying something new at a restaurant, let yourself enjoy the hell out of it.

Step eight: redefine what health means to you. Diet culture has hijacked the word "health" and turned it into a euphemism for thinness. But health is so much more than that. It's about feeling good in your body, having energy, and being able to do the things you love. It's about mental and emotional well-being, not just physical fitness. Your food philosophy should reflect your definition of health, not diet culture's bullshit version.

Step nine: be kind to yourself. Creating your own food philosophy doesn't mean you'll get it right every time. There will be days when you overeat, days when you under-eat, and days when you eat nothing but chips and dip. And that's okay. Food freedom is not about being perfect—it's about being human. So cut yourself some slack, forgive yourself for your "mistakes," and keep moving forward.

Step ten: celebrate your wins, big and small. Maybe you ate a meal without feeling guilty for the first time in years. Maybe you listened to your body and stopped eating when you were full. Maybe you tried a new food and loved it. Whatever it is, take a moment to acknowledge and celebrate your progress. Food freedom is a journey, not a destination, and every step you take is worth celebrating.

Creating your own food philosophy is one of the most empowering things you can do for yourself. It's about taking back control from diet culture, rejecting its bullshit rules, and living your life on your own terms. So go ahead, make your own rules—and then break them. Because you're the boss of your plate, and you get to decide what food freedom looks like for you.

Chapter 9

Fuck the Food Police and Their Judgy Faces

Shutting Down Food Shamers: A Masterclass in Saying, "Mind Your Own Plate, Karen"

Let's talk about the Food Police—the self-appointed sheriffs of your eating habits who think it's their job to critique every bite you take. You know the type. They're the ones side-eyeing your plate at family dinners, commenting on your grocery cart in the checkout line, or sliding into your DMs with unsolicited advice about carbs. Fuck these people. Your food choices are none of their business, and it's time to tell them exactly where they can shove their opinions.

First, let's break down who the Food Police are and why they exist. These are the people who've internalized diet culture so deeply that they feel the need to enforce its bullshit rules on everyone around them. They're the ones who've memorized the calorie count of every item on the Cheesecake Factory menu and can't wait to tell you about it. They're the ones who think ordering a salad makes them morally superior to you and your plate of nachos. Basically, they're the Karens of the culinary world, and they need to be stopped.

The Food Police come in many forms. There's the Concern Troll, who hides their judgment behind a thin veneer of faux compassion. "Oh, you're having dessert? I thought you were trying to lose weight!" Then there's the Holier-Than-Thou Health Nut, who thinks their green juice and kale chips make them better than you. "I could never eat something so unhealthy—it's all about balance, you know?" And let's not forget the Passive-Aggressive Prick, who delivers their critiques with a side of snark. "Wow, you must really love carbs!"

The common thread with all these assholes is that they think your food choices are up for debate. Spoiler alert: they're not. Your plate is not a community project, and you don't owe anyone an explanation for what you're eating. The Food Police can mind their own fucking business, and if they won't, it's time to clap back.

So how do you shut down food shamers without losing your cool (or your appetite)? First, let's talk about boundaries. Boundaries are the kryptonite of the Food Police—they hate them because boundaries make it clear that their opinions are neither wanted nor welcome. The next time someone tries to comment on your food, hit them with a simple, firm response: "I didn't ask for your opinion." Or, if you're feeling spicy, "You can worry about your plate, and I'll worry about mine."

If someone keeps pushing, don't be afraid to escalate. "Why are you so interested in what I'm eating? Is it because your own life is boring, or are you just a nosy asshole?" A little bit of humor goes a long way here—laughing at them takes away their power and makes it clear that you're not taking their bullshit seriously.

Let's also talk about dealing with the Food Police in social settings, because they love to show up uninvited to parties, dinners, and other group meals. These situations can be tricky, especially if the food shamer is someone you can't easily avoid, like a family member or coworker. In these cases, it's all about redirecting the conversation. "Wow, you seem really interested in what I'm eating. Maybe we should talk about something more interesting, like literally anything else."

If the Food Police start bringing up diet culture talking points—"Carbs are bad for you," "Sugar is the devil," "Are you sure you should be eating that?"—feel free to hit them with some cold, hard truth bombs. "Actually, carbs are a necessary source of energy for your body, and sugar isn't poison—it's just another type of food. Maybe you should do some research before spouting off bullshit." Or, if you want to keep it short and sweet, "Wow, that's a lot of misinformation in one sentence. Congrats!"

Sometimes, the Food Police will try to frame their comments as "helpful advice." Don't fall for it. "I'm just looking out for you" is code for "I think I know better than you." Shut that shit down with a clear statement of autonomy: "I appreciate your concern, but I'm perfectly capable of making my own decisions about what I eat."

And let's not forget about the Food Police on social media, because these assholes love to hide behind their keyboards. Whether it's a snarky comment on your food photo or an unsolicited DM about "clean eating," the best way to deal with online food shamers is to block, delete, and move the fuck on. You don't owe them your time, energy, or a debate.

Dealing with the Food Police can be exhausting, but it's important to remember that their judgment says more about them than it does about you. People who are secure in their own choices don't feel the need to police anyone else's. The Food Police are projecting their own insecurities, fears, and diet culture brainwashing onto you—and that's their problem, not yours.

Food freedom means refusing to let the Food Police control your plate, your choices, or your happiness. It means standing up for yourself, setting boundaries, and reminding these assholes that their opinions are not required or appreciated. So the next time someone tries to judge your food, take a deep breath, smile, and say, "Mind your own fucking plate, Karen." Then go back to enjoying your meal, because you deserve it.

Redefining Healthy: Spoiler: It Doesn't Mean Hating Yourself Into Submission

Let's get one thing straight: the word "healthy" has been hijacked. Diet culture swooped in, slapped a thin, airbrushed sticker on it, and turned it into a weapon of mass self-loathing. "Healthy" now means eating like a rabbit, working out until you puke, and pretending you enjoy kale chips more than actual chips. But here's the truth: real health isn't about punishing yourself or fitting into some bullshit societal standard. It's about feeling good in your body and your mind—no self-hatred required.

For too long, we've been sold the idea that health and thinness are the same thing. Spoiler alert: they're not. You can be thin and unhealthy, just like you can be fat and fit as fuck. Health isn't a size, a weight, or a look—it's a feeling. It's about energy, strength, and balance, not about squeezing into a pair of jeans from high school. And let's be real: those jeans were ugly as hell anyway.

The first step in redefining healthy is unlearning all the diet culture bullshit you've been force-fed over the years. Forget everything you've heard about "clean eating," detoxes, and "earning" your food. Real health isn't about restriction—it's about nourishment. It's about giving your body what it needs, whether that's a salad, a slice of cake, or a nap. It's about finding a balance that works for you, not for some Instagram influencer with a sponsorship deal.

Let's talk about exercise, because diet culture has completely fucked up our relationship with movement. Instead of being something we do for fun, stress relief, or strength, exercise has become a form of punishment—a way to "make up" for eating or to "earn" our calories. Fuck that. Movement should be joyful, not a chore. Whether it's dancing, hiking, swimming, or lifting heavy shit, find something you love and do it because it feels good, not because you're trying to "fix" yourself.

Health is also about mental well-being, which diet culture conveniently forgets. You can eat all the kale in the world, but if you're constantly stressed, anxious, and hating yourself, you're not healthy. Mental health is just as important as physical health, and sometimes that means eating comfort food, skipping the gym, or saying "fuck it" and watching Netflix all day. Taking care of your mind is just as valid as taking care of your body, and anyone who tells you otherwise can fuck right off.

Redefining healthy also means letting go of the idea that you have to be perfect. Diet culture thrives on this all-or-nothing mentality, where you're either a health god or a lazy slob with no willpower. But health isn't black and white—it's a spectrum. Some days you'll eat veggies and go for a run; other days you'll eat pizza and binge reality TV. Both days are valid, and neither one defines your worth.

One of the most toxic ideas diet culture pushes is that you have to hate yourself to be healthy. "Use your flaws as motivation!" they say. "Change your body to love your body!" they scream. But here's the thing: self-hatred is not a sustainable fuel source. You can't hate yourself into health, happiness, or anything else worth having. True health starts with self-acceptance, not self-loathing.

Self-acceptance doesn't mean giving up or settling—it means treating yourself with kindness and respect, no matter where you are in your journey. It means recognizing that your body is doing its best to keep you alive and that you don't need to punish it for not looking like a fitness model. It means appreciating what your body can do instead of obsessing over what it looks like.

Another key part of redefining healthy is rejecting the idea that health is a competition. Diet culture loves to turn health into a pissing contest, where everyone's comparing their macros, step counts, and gym selfies. But real health isn't about impressing anyone else—it's about taking care of yourself in a way that feels right for you. You don't need to prove your health to anyone, and you sure as hell don't need to compete with Karen and her keto recipes.

Let's also talk about food, because diet culture has completely fucked up our relationship with it. Food is not the enemy, and eating isn't a crime. Your body needs food to survive, and you deserve to enjoy it without guilt or fear. Real health isn't about obsessing over every bite you take—it's about nourishing your body and your soul.

Nourishment looks different for everyone. For some people, it's a colorful plate of veggies and lean protein. For others, it's a big-ass bowl of pasta with extra cheese. Both are valid, and both can be part of a healthy lifestyle. The key is listening to your body, honoring your cravings, and finding a balance that works for you.

Redefining healthy also means setting boundaries with the people and messages that don't support your journey. If someone is constantly shaming your choices, offering unsolicited advice, or trying to push their diet culture bullshit on you, it's okay to shut that shit down. Your health is your business, and you don't owe anyone an explanation for how you choose to take care of yourself.

Finally, remember that health is a journey, not a destination. There's no finish line, no perfect end point where you've "made it." Health is a lifelong practice of listening to your body, adapting to its needs, and finding joy in the process. It's not about being perfect—it's about being kind to yourself, every step of the way.

Redefining healthy means taking back the word from diet culture and making it your own. It means rejecting the idea that health is about thinness, perfection, or punishment, and embracing a new definition that prioritizes nourishment, balance, and self-love. So fuck the rules, fuck the guilt, and fuck the diet culture bullshit. You're in charge of your health, and you get to define what that means.

Owning Your Food Choices: Yes, I'm Having Fries and a Milkshake—Deal With It

Let's cut the bullshit: you don't owe anyone an explanation for what you eat. Not your mom, not your judgy coworker, and definitely not

Karen from HR who won't shut the fuck up about her "clean eating journey." Your food choices are yours, and you don't need to apologize, justify, or make excuses for them. Want fries and a milkshake? Own it. Love a big-ass plate of nachos? Go for it. Life is too fucking short to worry about what other people think about what's on your plate.

Here's the thing: diet culture has brainwashed us into thinking we have to defend our food choices. If you're eating something indulgent, you're supposed to tack on a self-deprecating comment like, "Oh, I'll be good tomorrow." If you're eating something "healthy," you're expected to explain how virtuous and disciplined you are. Fuck that. Food isn't a moral decision, and you don't owe anyone a play-by-play of why you're eating what you're eating.

Let's talk about the guilt that diet culture loves to sprinkle on everything, like a shitty seasoning nobody asked for. The moment you order fries, it creeps in: "Should I have gotten the salad? Am I going to regret this later? What will people think?" But here's the truth: guilt doesn't belong at the table. Guilt doesn't make your food taste better, nourish your body, or contribute anything positive to your life. It's just a waste of mental energy, and it's time to kick it to the curb.

Owning your food choices means letting go of the need for approval. You don't need a permission slip to enjoy dessert or a pat on the back for eating a salad. Your plate is yours, and it doesn't require anyone else's input. The next time someone raises an eyebrow at your order, try this: take a slow, deliberate bite, look them dead in the eye, and say, "Damn, this is good." Watch them squirm while you enjoy every fucking second of it.

Let's also address the people who feel the need to comment on your food choices, as if their unsolicited opinions are a gift to the world. "Oh, you're getting fries? I couldn't." Good for you, Karen. Nobody asked. "Wow, that's a lot of sugar." And wow, that's a lot of judgment for someone who isn't paying for my meal. These people thrive on making others feel small, and the best way to deal with them is to stand tall and unapologetic.

Owning your food choices isn't just about shutting down the haters—it's about embracing your cravings and trusting your body. If you want fries, it's because your body is craving something salty, crunchy, and satisfying. If you want a milkshake, it's because your body is saying, "Hey, let's enjoy something sweet and creamy right now." Your cravings aren't random—they're your body's way of communicating its needs. So listen to them and honor them without overthinking it.

Diet culture loves to make us second-guess our instincts, as if our bodies are these clueless assholes that can't be trusted. "Are you sure you're hungry? Maybe you're just thirsty." Fuck that noise. Your body is a genius, and it knows what it needs. The problem isn't your cravings—it's the bullshit narratives diet culture has planted in your head.

Owning your food choices also means letting go of the need to label foods as "good" or "bad." A milkshake isn't "bad," and a salad isn't "good." They're just different. Sometimes you want something light and fresh, and sometimes you want something rich and indulgent. Both are valid, and both can coexist in a balanced diet. The key is listening to your body and giving it what it needs in the moment.

Let's talk about balance, because diet culture loves to twist that word into something restrictive and joyless. True balance isn't about eating a kale salad so you can "earn" a slice of pizza—it's about giving yourself the freedom to enjoy all foods without guilt or judgment. It's about recognizing that fries and milkshakes have just as much of a place in your diet as fruits and veggies.

Owning your food choices also means standing firm in the face of societal pressure. We live in a world that glorifies thinness, discipline, and self-control, while shaming indulgence, pleasure, and joy. But here's the thing: you don't have to play by society's fucked-up rules. You're allowed to prioritize your happiness, satisfaction, and well-being over someone else's idea of what you "should" eat.

If you're struggling to own your food choices, start small. The next time you order something indulgent, resist the urge to make a self-deprecating comment or seek validation from others. Instead, focus on enjoying your food and reminding yourself that you have every right to eat it. With practice, this confidence will become second nature, and you'll stop giving a fuck about what anyone else thinks.

Owning your food choices is about reclaiming your autonomy and rejecting diet culture's bullshit. It's about trusting your body, embracing your cravings, and living your life unapologetically. So the next time someone questions your order, take a deep breath, smile, and say, "Yes, I'm having fries and a milkshake. Deal with it." Then savor every fucking bite, because you deserve it.

Chapter 10

Celebrate Every Damn Bite

Food Is Love, Joy, and Culture: Not Just Fuel for Your Gym Grind

Let's be real—food isn't just fuel. It's not some joyless equation of calories in and calories out. Food is love, connection, celebration, and, yes, sometimes a coping mechanism when life feels like one big flaming shitshow. And you know what? That's okay. It's time to stop thinking of food as just a means to an end and start treating it like the delicious, soul-nourishing gift that it is. Every bite you take is a moment worth celebrating, and it's about damn time you started acting like it.

Diet culture loves to strip food of its magic. "Food is fuel," they say, as if a plate of tacos is the same as pumping gas into your car. But here's the thing: you're not a fucking car. You're a human being with taste buds, emotions, and a deep, primal need for joy. Food isn't just about survival—it's about thriving. It's about savoring a perfectly crispy French fry, indulging in a rich slice of cheesecake, and sharing a home-cooked meal with the people you love.

Food is love, plain and simple. It's your grandma's lasagna, made with enough cheese to clog an artery and enough love to heal a broken heart. It's your best friend baking you a cake for your birthday, even though they know you're not a "cake person." It's your partner bringing you takeout after a shitty day because they know exactly what you need to feel human again. Food is how we care for each other, and reducing it to a number on a nutrition label completely misses the point.

Food is also joy—the kind of joy that makes you close your eyes and let out an involuntary "mmm" when you take that first bite. It's the joy of biting into a perfectly juicy burger, the kind that drips down your hands and makes you regret not grabbing extra napkins. It's the joy of sneaking a spoonful of cookie dough before it even makes it to the oven. It's the joy of indulging in something purely because it tastes good, with no guilt or shame attached.

And let's not forget that food is culture—a way of preserving our histories, traditions, and identities. It's your mom's famous holiday cookies, your family's secret BBQ recipe, or that one dish that only your dad can get right. It's street food in a foreign city, tasting flavors you've never experienced before. It's a potluck with friends, where every dish tells a story. Food connects us to our roots, our communities, and the world around us.

But diet culture doesn't give a fuck about any of that. It reduces food to macros, calories, and portion sizes, stripping away everything that makes it meaningful. It tells you to eat the grilled chicken instead of the fried, to skip dessert, and to say no to seconds. It takes something sacred and turns it into a source of stress and shame. And it's time to call bullshit.

Celebrating every bite starts with letting go of the guilt. Guilt is diet culture's favorite weapon, and it serves no purpose other than to make you miserable. You didn't "cheat" by eating a cookie, and you're not "bad" for having seconds. Food is not a test of your morality, and you don't need to pass some imaginary exam to enjoy it. The next time guilt creeps in, tell it to fuck off and focus on the joy of what you're eating.

Celebration also means slowing the fuck down and savoring your food. Diet culture has us so obsessed with rules and restrictions that we barely even taste what we're eating. We're too busy counting calories, logging macros, and planning our next meal to enjoy the one in front of us. But food deserves your full attention. Take a bite, close your eyes, and really taste it. Notice the flavors, the textures, and the way it makes you feel. This isn't about being "mindful" in some preachy, yoga-teacher way—it's about giving food the respect it fucking deserves.

Part of celebrating every bite is sharing it with others. Food is inherently communal—it's meant to be enjoyed together, whether it's a fancy dinner party or a late-night run to Taco Bell. Sharing a meal with someone is one of the most intimate, human things you can do. It's a way of saying, "I care about you enough to let you see me with sauce on my face and crumbs in my lap." So break bread with the people you love, and let the joy of connection elevate your experience.

Celebrating food also means embracing its imperfections. Not every meal has to be Instagram-worthy or meticulously plated. Some of the best food comes from a greasy diner, a backyard BBQ, or your kitchen at 2 a.m. when you're just throwing shit together. Food doesn't have to be fancy to be meaningful—it just has to be real.

Another way to celebrate food is to honor its role in your life. Food isn't just about taste—it's about memories, emotions, and experiences. It's the Thanksgiving dinners that turned into family stories, the first meal you cooked for someone you loved, or the midnight snacks that got you through a tough time. Food is woven into the fabric of our lives, and it deserves to be celebrated for everything it represents.

Finally, celebrating every bite means letting go of perfection. You don't have to eat "clean" to be healthy, and you don't have to follow anyone else's rules to enjoy your food. Eat what makes you happy, and eat it unapologetically. Whether it's a kale salad or a double cheeseburger, every bite is worth celebrating because it's part of your unique, messy, beautiful life.

Food is so much more than fuel for your gym grind. It's love, joy, culture, and connection. It's a way of caring for yourself and others, of honoring your past and creating new memories. So stop letting diet culture steal the joy from your plate. Celebrate every damn bite, and live your life with the kind of flavor it deserves.

Cheers to Progress: Reflecting on Your Journey to Giving Zero F*cks About Diets

Let's take a moment to raise a glass (or a donut) and toast to how far you've come. Seriously, cheers to you. Whether you've burned your diet books, told Karen from HR to mind her own fucking plate, or just ordered fries without a side of guilt for the first time in years, you're making progress. And that shit deserves to be celebrated. This is your journey to giving zero fucks about diets, and you're killing it.

Think about where you started. Maybe you were knee-deep in the bullshit, obsessing over carbs, counting every calorie, and measuring out portions like you were preparing for a NASA mission. Maybe you were the person who packed a sad salad to every barbecue or skipped dessert at your own birthday party. You were stuck in the diet culture hamster wheel, chasing an impossible ideal and hating yourself every step of the way. And then something clicked.

At some point, you realized that diets were never going to give you the happiness or self-worth they promised. Maybe it was a lightbulb moment, or maybe it was a slow burn—a nagging feeling that there had to be a better way. Whatever it was, it brought you here, to this moment of reflection, where you can finally see the progress you've made. And damn, is it worth celebrating.

The first step on this journey was probably the hardest: giving yourself permission to eat what the fuck you want. Diet culture had you so deep in its clutches that even thinking about pizza felt like a rebellion. But you did it. You started listening to your cravings, honoring your hunger, and trusting your body. You stopped letting the fear of food control your life, and that's a big fucking deal.

Then you started setting boundaries. You told the Food Police to back the fuck off. You stopped explaining, justifying, and apologizing for your food choices. You reclaimed your plate and your power, and you started eating on your own terms. That's some badass shit right there.

You also learned how to quiet the loudmouth in your head—the one that diet culture planted there to judge and shame you every time you ate something "bad." You stopped letting that voice run the show, and you replaced it with compassion, curiosity, and a whole lot of sass. You started talking back, saying things like, "No, I'm not going to feel guilty for eating a cupcake," and "Yes, I'm going to have seconds because this mac and cheese is fucking delicious."

As you kept moving forward, you started seeing food for what it really is: nourishment, joy, and connection. You stopped treating it like a moral test or a punishment, and you started celebrating it instead. You savored every bite, shared meals with the people you love, and found joy in the simple act of eating.

You also learned how to navigate the bullshit. You figured out how to spot diet culture's sneaky tactics—the guilt-language, the "wellness" disguises, the unsolicited advice—and you shut that shit down. You stopped falling for the traps, and you started living your life without the constant shadow of food fear.

And let's not forget the most important part of this journey: you stopped giving a fuck. You stopped caring what other people think about your food choices. You stopped worrying about whether you were eating "the right way." You stopped letting diet culture dictate your life. You found freedom, and it looks damn good on you.

Of course, the journey hasn't been perfect. There have been setbacks, moments of doubt, and days when the old habits crept back in. But progress isn't about perfection—it's about persistence. Every time you chose self-love over self-loathing, every time you celebrated a meal instead of fearing it, every time you stood up to diet culture, you took another step forward. And that's what matters.

So where do you go from here? Wherever the fuck you want. This is your life, your journey, and your plate. You've proven that you're capable of breaking free from the bullshit, and now it's time to keep building on that progress. Keep listening to your body, setting boundaries, and celebrating every bite. Keep living your life unapologetically, with zero fucks given about diets or anyone else's opinions.

Remember that this journey isn't about reaching some final destination. There's no finish line, no gold star, no moment when you'll have it all figured out. It's a lifelong process of learning, growing, and evolving. Some days will be easier than others, and that's okay. What matters is that you keep showing up for yourself, every damn day.

And when you do stumble—because let's face it, you're human, and it's going to happen—be kind to yourself. There's no such thing as failure on this journey, only opportunities to learn and grow. So pick yourself up, dust yourself off, and keep moving forward. You've got this.

As you reflect on how far you've come, take a moment to appreciate the badass that you are. You've done the hard work of unlearning diet culture's bullshit, reclaiming your relationship with food, and finding your own version of freedom. That's no small feat, and it deserves to be celebrated. So raise a glass, a slice of cake, or a double cheeseburger, and toast to your progress.

Cheers to you, and cheers to the rest of your journey. Here's to living your life with joy, balance, and absolutely zero fucks given about diets. You're a badass, and don't you forget it.

Your New Normal: Living a Guilt-Free, Food-Filled Life Like the Badass You Are

Welcome to your new normal: a life where food isn't a source of stress, shame, or self-loathing, but a source of joy, connection, and unapologetic indulgence. Gone are the days of calorie counting, food rules, and apologizing for your choices. You're officially living the dream—a guilt-free, food-filled life like the badass you are. And let me tell you, it looks fucking fantastic on you.

Living guilt-free starts with embracing the fact that you're not perfect—and you don't have to be. Diet culture loves to sell the illusion of perfection, promising happiness and self-worth if you just eat clean enough, thin enough, or "right" enough. But here's the thing: perfection is bullshit. It's unattainable, unsustainable, and completely unnecessary. Your new normal isn't about being perfect—it's about being real.

Real means eating a balanced breakfast one day and cold pizza the next. It means hitting the gym because you want to, not because you feel like you have to "earn" your dinner. It means indulging in dessert without a second thought or skipping it because you're just not in the mood. Real is messy, imperfect, and full of contradictions—and that's what makes it beautiful.

Your new normal also means making peace with your cravings. Cravings are not the enemy, and they're not a test of your willpower. They're your body's way of saying, "Hey, I could really go for some chocolate right now," or "How about some fries to make this day suck a little less?" Instead of fighting your cravings, you've learned to honor them, trust them, and enjoy the hell out of whatever you're craving.

Part of living a guilt-free, food-filled life is shutting down the voices—both internal and external—that try to rain on your parade. Whether it's the diet culture gremlin in your head or the Food Police at the table next to you, you've gotten damn good at telling them to fuck off. Your food choices are yours and yours alone, and you don't owe anyone an explanation.

Your new normal means saying yes to the bread basket, the dessert menu, and the late-night drive-thru runs. It means saying no to guilt, shame, and unsolicited advice. It means eating for pleasure, for nourishment, and sometimes just because you fucking feel like it. It's about reclaiming food as a source of joy and connection, not a battlefield.

Speaking of connection, your new normal also means enjoying food as a shared experience. It's not just about what's on your plate—it's about who you're eating it with. It's about Sunday brunch with friends, family dinners filled with laughter, and late-night snacks shared with someone who gets you. Food has always been a way to bring people together, and now you're finally letting it play that role in your life without the interference of diet culture's bullshit.

Living guilt-free doesn't mean throwing balance out the window—it means redefining what balance looks like for you. Balance isn't a rigid set of rules or a perfect ratio of "good" to "bad" foods. It's a fluid, flexible concept that changes based on your needs, cravings, and circumstances. Some days, balance might mean a kale smoothie and a quinoa salad. Other days, it might mean a burger and fries with a side of chocolate cake. Both days are valid, and both are part of your new normal.

Your new normal also means letting go of the need to "fix" yourself. Diet culture thrives on convincing us that we're broken—that we're not thin enough, disciplined enough, or worthy enough. But you've realized that's all a load of shit. You're not broken, and you don't need fixing.

You're a badass just as you are, and your worth isn't tied to your weight, your diet, or your fitness routine.

Part of living a guilt-free life is embracing your body as it is, not as you think it "should" be. That doesn't mean you have to love every inch of yourself every second of every day—because, let's be real, who does? It means treating your body with kindness, respect, and gratitude, even on the days when you're not feeling your best. It means recognizing that your body is doing its best to keep you alive, and that's pretty fucking amazing.

Your new normal means celebrating food in all its forms. It's about savoring the rich, indulgent meals as much as the simple, nourishing ones. It's about appreciating the cultural, emotional, and sensory experiences that food brings to your life. It's about treating every bite as an opportunity to connect with yourself, your loved ones, and the world around you.

Living guilt-free doesn't mean you'll never have moments of doubt or insecurity—because you will. There will still be days when diet culture tries to sneak back in, whispering its bullshit into your ear. But the difference now is that you know how to shut it down. You know how to remind yourself that you're in control, not diet culture. And you know how to keep moving forward, even when the old habits try to creep back in.

Your new normal isn't just about food—it's about freedom. Freedom from the rules, the guilt, and the endless cycle of self-loathing. Freedom to eat what you want, when you want, without apology or explanation. Freedom to live your life on your own terms, with zero fucks given about what anyone else thinks.

So here's to you and your new normal. Here's to living a guilt-free, food-filled life like the badass you are. Here's to fries and milkshakes, Sunday brunches, and midnight snacks. Here's to saying fuck you to diet culture and hello to food freedom. Because you've earned it, you deserve it, and you're fucking rocking it.

100 Fuck Dieting Tips to Live Your Best Food-Filled Life

Welcome to the part of the book where we break it all down—no fluff, no bullshit, just real talk. These tips are your guide to living a guilt-free, food-filled life without the shackles of diet culture weighing you down. Whether you need a reminder to eat the damn cake, tell Karen to mind her business, or just embrace the joy of food again, this list has you covered. Each tip is a little nugget of wisdom (and sass) to help you reclaim your plate, your peace, and your power. So dig in and get ready to say, "Fuck dieting!" for good.

Tip #1
Stop labeling foods as "good" or "bad." Food doesn't have morals, and neither does your plate.

Tip #2
Eat the damn bread. Life is too short to skip the bread basket.

Tip #3
Ignore calorie counts on menus—they're a buzzkill and don't belong at the table.

Tip #4

Trust your cravings. If you're craving chocolate, eat the chocolate.

Tip #5

Celebrate every bite. Food is joy, not a punishment.

Tip #6

Throw out the scale. Your worth isn't measured in pounds.

Tip #7

Say no to "cheat days." You don't need permission to enjoy food.

Tip #8

Stop apologizing for your food choices. You don't owe anyone an explanation.

Tip #9

Make peace with carbs. They're not the enemy—they're delicious.

Tip #10

Listen to your body. It knows what it needs better than diet culture does.

Tip #11

Savor your food. Eating isn't a race—it's an experience.

Tip #12

Stop trying to "earn" your food with exercise. Eat because you're hungry, not because you burned calories.

Tip #13

Set boundaries with food shamers. Your plate, your rules.

Tip #14

Indulge in dessert. Life is sweeter when you don't skip the cake.

Tip #15

Ditch the guilt. You're not "bad" for eating a donut.

Tip #16

Don't skip meals to "save calories." That's diet culture bullshit.

Tip #17

Unfollow accounts that make you feel bad about your body or your food choices.

Tip #18

Treat food as a source of connection and culture, not just fuel.

Tip #19

Trust your hunger cues. If you're hungry, eat.

Tip #20

Learn to love leftovers. They're a delicious reminder of yesterday's joy.

Tip #21

Stop fearing fat in your diet. Fat is flavor, and your body needs it.

Tip #22

Celebrate non-scale wins, like enjoying your favorite meal guilt-free.

Tip #23

Don't overthink your portions. Eat until you're satisfied, not stuffed.

Tip #24

Be unapologetically indulgent. Order the fries and the milkshake.

Tip #25

Embrace imperfection. Not every meal has to be "healthy."

Tip #26

Focus on progress, not perfection. Every step toward food freedom is worth celebrating.

Tip #27

Cook for joy, not just nutrition. A little butter won't kill you.

Tip #28

Practice saying, "Mind your own plate," when people comment on your food.

Tip #29

Stop comparing your plate to others. Your journey is your own.

Tip #30

Rediscover your favorite childhood snacks. Nostalgia tastes amazing.

Tip #31

Drink your calories if you want to. Milkshakes, juice, and wine are valid choices.

Tip #32

Embrace second helpings if you're still hungry. Your body knows what it needs.

Tip #33

Forget "clean eating." Food doesn't need to be sanitized for approval.

Tip #34

Say yes to pizza night. Balance is about joy, not deprivation.

Tip #35

Learn to enjoy eating alone. Your company is enough.

Tip #36

Eat what makes you happy, not what someone else thinks you should eat.

Tip #37

Throw out the detox teas. Your liver is already a detox machine.

Tip #38

Don't let diet culture ruin holidays. Enjoy the food, guilt-free.

Tip #39

Practice gratitude for your body and the food that nourishes it.

Tip #40

Order the burger instead of the salad if that's what you really want.

Tip #41

Stop skipping carbs at dinner. They help you sleep better.

Tip #42

Say goodbye to portion control. Listen to your body instead.

Tip #43

Stop obsessing over "healthy swaps." Sometimes you just want the real thing.

Tip #44

Learn to laugh at diet culture. It's ridiculous, and it deserves to be mocked.

Tip #45

Choose joy over macros. You won't remember the calorie count, but you'll remember the experience.

Tip #46

Share meals with loved ones. Food tastes better with good company.

Tip #47

Embrace midnight snacks. Hunger doesn't follow a schedule.

Tip #48

Forget "summer bodies." Your body is already perfect for summer.

Tip #49

Say yes to butter. It's delicious, and your toast deserves it.

Tip #50

Practice food neutrality. A donut is no better or worse than a salad.

Tip #51

Throw away the meal prep containers if they stress you out.

Tip #52

Eat the ice cream straight from the tub. It's called efficiency.

Tip #53

Stop fearing sodium. Your body needs it to survive.

Tip #54

Reclaim brunch as a guilt-free celebration.

Tip #55

Trust your full signals. Stop eating when you're satisfied, not stuffed.

Tip #56

Order appetizers without shame. They're meant to be enjoyed.

Tip #57

Say goodbye to "low-fat" labels. Flavor is your friend.

Tip #58

Enjoy food without multitasking. Sit down and savor it.

Tip #59

Stop apologizing for your cravings. They're valid and normal.

Tip #60

Say yes to food adventures. Try the weird dish on the menu.

Tip #61

Honor your traditions. Cultural foods are sacred, not "cheat meals."

Tip #62

Eat what's in front of you without worrying about the next meal.

Tip #63

Stop demonizing sugar. It's just a carbohydrate, not Satan.

Tip #64

Learn to say, "No, thanks," to diet talk at the table.

Tip #65

Pack snacks you love, not just ones that seem "healthy."

Tip #66

Stop obsessing over labels. Gluten-free doesn't mean guilt-free.

Tip #67

Redefine comfort food. It's called comfort for a reason.

Tip #68

Say yes to dessert first, if that's what you're craving.

Tip #69

Be unapologetic about food that makes you happy.

Tip #70

Eat at restaurants without checking the menu first.

Tip #71

Stop punishing yourself for eating "too much."

Tip #72

Learn to say, "Fuck it," and enjoy the meal.

Tip #73

Cook without measuring everything. Trust your instincts.

Tip #74

Enjoy the taste of real butter, sugar, and cream.

Tip #75

Don't let anyone shame you for eating fast food.

Tip #76

Let your food choices reflect your mood, not someone else's rules.

Tip #77

Stop skipping breakfast to "save calories."

Tip #78

Rediscover the joy of baking and eating your creations.

Tip #79

Learn to say yes to cravings without guilt.

Tip #80

Reclaim food as a celebration, not a chore.

Tip #81

Ditch the apps that track your meals.

Tip #82

Let go of food fear. Eating isn't dangerous—it's essential.

Tip #83

Stop trying to "hack" your diet. Just eat the food.

Tip #84

Learn to love your food choices, no matter what they are.

Tip #85

Stop worrying about your plate being "balanced."

Tip #86

Say no to "cleanse" culture.

Tip #87

Celebrate indulgent meals as part of a balanced life.

Tip #88

Eat what you love, even if it's not "trendy."

Tip #89

Stop following restrictive diets that steal your joy.

Tip #90

Say yes to spontaneous food decisions.

Tip #91

Relearn the joy of eating without a plan.

Tip #92

Enjoy food for what it is, not what it "should" be.

Tip #93

Stop treating food as a transaction.

Tip #94

Celebrate your progress toward food freedom.

Tip #95

Make every meal a moment to enjoy.

Tip #96

Forget the rules and listen to your body.

Tip #97

Rediscover the pleasure of eating for fun.

Tip #98

Reclaim food as a source of joy, not stress.

Tip #99

Learn to trust yourself around all foods.

Tip #100

Eat the fucking cake. You deserve it.

Here's to Living Your Best, Most Delicious Life

You made it! You've officially given diet culture the middle finger and reclaimed your relationship with food. Whether you're indulging in fries without a side of guilt, savoring a late-night slice of pizza, or unapologetically rocking your body just as it is, you've taken a massive step toward food freedom. And damn, doesn't it feel good?

This journey wasn't about following someone else's rules—it was about smashing those rules to bits and writing your own. It was about unlearning the toxic bullshit diet culture has been spewing and discovering what truly makes you feel happy, nourished, and alive. It's about embracing balance, not perfection, and finding joy in every bite you take.

So where do you go from here? Wherever the fuck you want. Your plate is yours to fill with whatever makes you happy—be it nachos, kale, or both at the same time. You've learned to trust your cravings, listen to your body, and silence the noise of guilt and shame. That's a level of badassery most people only dream of achieving.

But remember, this journey doesn't end here. It's a lifelong process of learning, growing, and continuing to tell diet culture to fuck off. There will be challenges—moments when the old habits try to creep back in, or when someone's unsolicited opinion threatens to ruin your vibe. But now, you've got the tools, the confidence, and the attitude to handle it like the badass you are.

So here's to you and your food freedom. Here's to meals that bring joy, laughter, and connection. Here's to loving your body without conditions and living your life without restrictions. Here's to fries, milkshakes, and everything else that makes your soul happy.

Now go out there and live your best, most delicious life. You've earned it, you deserve it, and the world is a better (and tastier) place with you in it. Cheers!

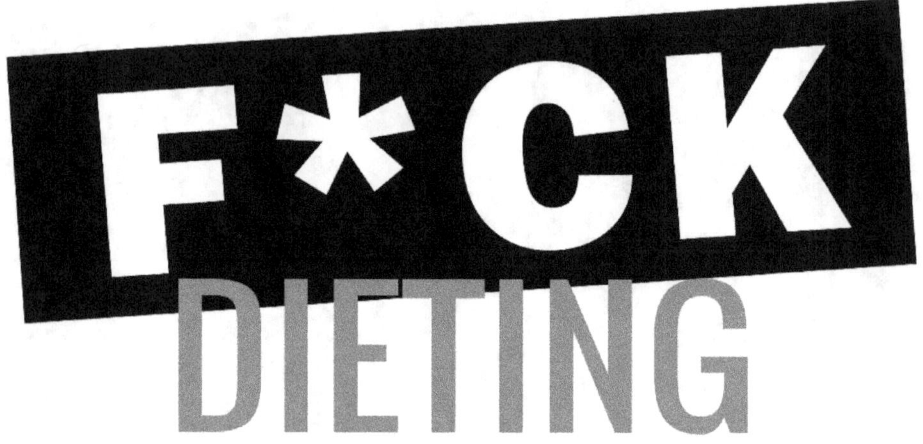

The Badass Guide to Smashing Diet Culture One F*cking Bite at a Time!

Logan West